Living With Depression
Journeys to Healing

Leanne Warr

Living With Depression
Journeys to Healing

Living with depression is not easy. It can make you moody and sometimes impossible to live with. It's hard enough for the person with this illness, but just as hard on family members who have no idea how to deal with it.

For some, depression can have devastating consequences.

Over 300 million people in the world have been diagnosed with this illness, yet there are still those out there who have no knowledge or understanding of it and how debilitating it can be.

I have struggled for years with the effects of depression, bullying and emotional abuse. There are others like me who have been through something similar and we are only now coming out the other side.

This book is not just my own journey. It seeks to explain what depression is while dispelling the myths around it and what causes it through research and personal analysis.

I also include some coping strategies - some I have experienced personally and others through extensive research.

Above all, I believe there is a way to heal.

Dedication and Acknowledgements

For Kat, who has helped me navigate my way through this journey. Without your invaluable help, I would never have got this far.

For Carol, Meg and Mum, for all you have put up with.

For Jenny. There are no words to describe how much you have been there for me in my darkest moments.

Thank you to those who have provided some insight and been kind enough to allow me to borrow their expertise. And to those who have told their own stories, your input has been invaluable.

AUTHOR'S NOTE

Where possible, I have gained feedback from writers of various articles in order to present some research background. Some of the articles mentioned are from online magazines or websites.

Thanks to the following: Professor Mark Humphries, Dr Taylor Chastain, Dr Stephen Diamond, Dr Sarah Gingell, Dr Joseph Firth and the staff at the NICM Health Research Institute Dr David Hill and Professor Anthony Campbell. Also to the NZ Ministry of Health, the National Institute of Mental Health (US), the World Health Organisation, Beyond Blue, the *New Zealand Herald*, the *New York Times*, *Psychology Today* and all other organisations who made their publications available via the Internet which was invaluable to my research.

Articles and websites used are referenced in the Bibliography. Please do visit these sites for further reading.

Foreword

I asked one of the people I interviewed in this book to write some thoughts as a precede to our stories. I also asked my counsellor to add her thoughts.

Kathy

I have had a long-term association with depression, but this is only one aspect of my life. Depression has been accepted and relegated to a back corner; learn to live with your limitations and carry on.

To have someone that is warm, caring and ready to listen, that totally understands the impact depression has on your daily life is a relief and a release for those deeply suppressed emotions.

Depression is experienced in a variety of ways, different for every individual although there are common elements running through each story.

By expressing our own experience others can see there is no reason to be isolated, by sharing our own story hopefully this will open up dialogue and bring hope. That
it is OK to exist in our own bubble, but maybe we can push the boundaries just a little and extend our comfort zone.

We need to find our own solutions that work best; listen to advice and choose what fits our personality and lifestyle.

Remember there is no magical quick fix; takes acceptance, time and patience.

A support system is a bonus, the load is better shared around. Let others know what you need, find those that understand and can contribute positively to your life; accept the help that is offered.

Know that there will be great days, bad days, but each will pass. Just to live each day is progress; small steps are still moving forward, backwards is just a detour, just be patient. Always treat yourself with kindness and compassion, you are doing the best you can. Do something you enjoy daily.

For myself I require plenty of alone time, retreat into a world of books, limit my exposure to stressful situations and try to accept myself just as I am!

Kat Steeneken
AAMINZ, NZAFT, NZAPP, MANZASW, NZAC (Prov)

Leanne writes from the heart drawing on personal experience and strategies used to manage her own symptoms, learning what works for her.

Leanne makes the point that depression is a journey and its management is very personal.

The book is honest and down to earth, each chapter well researched and considered.

What I like the most about this book is that it is written from the perspective of someone who has struggled to find strategies that work that are simple and easy to follow without bogging you down with tasks.

Leanne shares her own journey and her own trials and tribulations, sharing what has worked well for her as she has travelled down the path of self-discovery.

Leanne does not offer any quick fixes nor does she offer false hope. She simply offers the things that she has tried and the things that research has suggested might work well.

I feel honoured to be sharing this very personal journey with Leanne and hope that you, the reader, find solace within the words and the suggestions put forward as an aid for you on your personal journey of managing your depressive symptoms.

PREFACE

A few years ago, I was a guest speaker at a meeting of a Masonic Lodge chapter in Hamilton, speaking to some of the wives about depression. One of the questions that kept coming up was, why does someone with this illness commit suicide? And how can a family come to terms with this?

Another question that is often asked is: why is it so prevalent now? There is no simple answer to this. Statistics can only give us so much information, relying on the accuracy of reporting. However, in some countries, the stigma of mental illness is too strong for people to seek help. Here in New Zealand, the numbers show that more women are diagnosed with depression than men, but that may not be accurate either.

Depression may seem to be on the rise now, compared to thirty or forty years ago, but how can we know for sure? For hundreds of years, those with this illness would have suffered in silence, fearing they would be thought to be mad. Even fifty years ago, this was a subject that was not talked about so openly as it is today.

Nowadays, health professionals have more tools available to diagnose such illnesses, and there is far more awareness. However, there is also a risk that it may be over-diagnosed where symptoms of depression may be signs of something else.

There are already a number of books on depression and anxiety out there, yet people are still as confused as ever. Those who have never experienced it may continue to feel depression is something that 'everyone deals with from time to time', and they fail to understand why many sufferers are hospitalised.

It's easy to dismiss depression as something people use for attention. Yet most people do not realise that for the sufferer, it can be extremely debilitating.

Most suicides can be attributed to depression. It's considered a selfish act and those left behind are at a loss to understand how their loved one could do something that selfish. We can only guess at what was going through that person's mind, but based on anecdotal evidence from various attempts, the sufferer is not thinking of those they're leaving behind. All they are thinking of is ending their own pain.

I can attest to some of this. Often, the negative thoughts that lead to suicidal ideations are those that tell us we're a burden on our families, and that they will be better off if we weren't around; that we deserve all the bad things that happen to us. Unfortunately, sometimes, the words of those we love are not enough to change that mindset.

In many cases, an attempt at suicide is an attempt to silence those negative thoughts.

***

According to the New Zealand Health Survey 2016-2017, about 16 per cent of New Zealand's population, or around 640,000 people, had been diagnosed with depression in their lifetime. This is by no means an accurate picture of the real scope of mental illness, of which depression is just one part.

The numbers are based on estimates which, of course, are now slightly out-of-date and do not account for some people who have either not been diagnosed or have not sought help from health services. There are many countries in the world where getting help is just not possible and getting an accurate picture of the true state of affairs is equally impossible.

I consider myself extremely lucky to live in a country that has a slightly better healthcare system, although, for many who also live below the poverty line, a visit to a GP becomes prohibitive. Subsidies may take care of some things, but not everything.

In other countries, particularly in the developing world, where things like war, famine and disease are an everyday problem, the scope of mental illness can never be measured, simply because there are not the facilities in order to do so. It is also important to note that in some cultures, mental illness is ignored or dismissed. Others may choose to hide it for their own reasons.

It was not so long ago, even in countries like the United States, mental illness was considered to be dangerous. Three or four hundred years ago, people who were 'different' were thought to be possessed. It is only in the last century or so that we have been able to understand it and treat it.

Depression cannot be seen. It does not show as a physical deformity. Author Henry Wadsworth Longfellow once said: "Every man has secret sorrows the world knows not, and often times we call a man cold when he is only sad."

It has been called a number of things over the last two or three hundred years: sadness, melancholy. It has been misdiagnosed, mis-represented, misunderstood and in many ways, feared.

A number of historical figures were known to have depression.

Famed writer Agatha Christie, who wrote such volumes as *Murder on the Orient Express*, may have had depressive episodes. Author Virginia Woolf had a mental illness. Nineteenth century US president, Abraham Lincoln was known for 'hypochondria' and episodes of melancholy. Winston Churchill talked about a 'black dog', Ernest Hemingway, Vincent van Gogh, Hans Christian Andersen, Raymond Chandler, Calvin Coolidge, Charles Darwin, F. Scott Fitzgerald,

Judy Garland, Herman Melville, Wolfgang Amadeus Mozart, Friedrich Nietzsche, Edgar Allan Poe, Jackson Pollock, Mark Twain, Tennessee Williams, to name a few, also shared this illness in common.

Some famous people in more recent times have also been diagnosed with this illness. In the past five years or more, we have been shocked to learn of deaths of various celebrities, most by their own hand. Yet, why should they be treated any differently to the average person also struggling with this illness?

Usually, when we hear of the death of someone famous, the main question on people's minds is: why? These people have had great success in their lives and everything to live for. While it's a fair question, it shows just how little people understand what this illness is.

Depression can be a barrier to success, but success is not necessarily a barrier to depression. The fact that people can get this illness in spite of any successes in their personal lives shows that depression can strike anyone. Sir John Kirwan, a well-known All Black, was diagnosed with depression at the peak of his career. He has taken what he has learnt from his illness to raise awareness.

Yet, it is still an illness much misunderstood: by our employers, our friends, even our families. I have heard of stories of people being denied jobs because of their mental health, yet depression does not preclude someone from being able to work.

There is a reason depression is called the 'invisible illness'. Imagine walking down the street and meeting about 20 people. They all smile at you as they pass by. Now look closer at those smiles. Does one of them seem to falter? Which one? Can you really tell?

This is the problem with depression. The symptoms do not usually show up as something obvious. I read something on social media, which is highly relevant, which basically said that if depression was as obvious as a physical illness or disability, people would not be so quick to judge.

I was diagnosed with depression at the age of 17 and still struggle with it after 30 years. I am not the only one.

I don't consider myself to be special, just someone who can put thoughts into words and create some semblance of a story. I guess that sets me apart from others who have other ways of dealing with it.

In my struggles, I have done a great deal of self-analysis. My research has taken me down many paths, some of them successful, some not so. My thirst for knowledge and my desire to understand my own illness has helped me deal with some of the worst of it. For me, my depression has been a very lonely experience, hence the desire to share some of what I have learnt and perhaps help someone else who, like me, has become a little lost in the fog of their own struggle.

This book is not just about my own journey. It's about every person going through these same struggles. It will include facts and figures, research, and explore alternatives to medication.

I do not have all the answers. What works for me may not work for someone else. However, I hope that by sharing my story and knowledge from professionals, it may help someone else find their own way.

Currently, there is no cure for depression. Whether that will happen in the immediate future is hard to say. Mental illness is costly for all health services and research into its causes and treatments, leading to a cure, may not happen in my lifetime.

I can only hope that the pathways I have taken will continue to help me manage my depression.

Section One – My Journey

The following are some poems I wrote which, to me, help describe some of the stages of my journey. I have published these on Facebook and on a social media website.

THE INNER CRITIC (AKA MY NEMESIS)

"You're stupid!" says my nemesis
As I shut my mouth
Embarrassed at my own idiocy

The words had spewed forth
Like verbal diarrhoea
A light panel in my brain flashing
"Malfunction, malfunction"
"Danger Will Robinson!"

My enemy laughing loudly in my head
Bringing up incidents long forgotten
Examples of past stupidity
Pointing at me, shouting "Nyah nyah"

Leaving me beating my head against the wall
Hoping to shut up that inner critic
Never quite succeeding

ANXIETY

It feels like a ten-tonne weight
And I can't breathe
Lying on my back
And I can't move

My body seems weightless
Floating through space
Ground control calling but
All communication broken

The phone rings
It's my mum calling
Worried because I won't answer
I can't answer

Anxiety has me in its grip
Icy tentacles holding me tight
And won't let me breathe
Won't let me up

Story of my life

DEPRESSION

Hello darkness my old friend
I think that's how the line went

It speaks of what you once were to me
My constant companion

And now here you are again
Just popping in for a visit you say

It's okay, you can stay for a while
Maybe a cup of tea
But you know you gotta go soon
I've got things to do

So go on, stay a little bit
No, you can't hold my hand
We've been down this road before
We both know it's a dead-end

You know where the door is

This last one is my favourite because it is where I feel I am
in my depression.

Chapter One: Introduction

"Gidday, Ugly."

You would think after 30 years those words wouldn't have the power over me that they once did, but I can still feel the shock of hearing them, see the guy walking across the street, staring at me as I cycled home from school. A man who really had nothing to write home about in the looks department yet could call out such an insult.

I had no idea who this man was and still don't. I was 15 years old. Skinny and short for my age. I was not a confident child. Shy and quiet, I would get red in the face if I was called on in class. I found the whole process terrifying.

I was the little mouse in school who preferred to sit in the corner and just do my work. There was no doubt I was reasonably gifted in the intelligence department, but my inability to communicate and my lack of confidence only produced average grades. I still managed to pass all my classes but very rarely made it to the top percentile of the class. That was reserved for those who were not lacking in self-confidence.

Was I ugly? I would hardly have called myself that, but that I can still recall those words means they continue to impact my life after all this time.

There is a saying: "Sticks and stones may break my bones, but words can never hurt me." Whoever came up with that saying is wrong. Words can, and do, hurt; as I have learnt through my experiences.

Another incident, around the same time, made me question what people thought of me. I was passing a girl who, from what I can recall, was the sister of a girl in my class. I was not friends with my classmate. To be honest, I didn't like her that much, not that I would have ever told her that. I tend to wear my heart on my sleeve, so to speak, and perhaps I projected my dislike for the girl.

As I passed the older girl, I heard her call out: "Slut!"

I still remember the shock through my body as I heard that word. I knew what it meant. I was not so naïve that I didn't understand terms like that. Why was she calling me a slut? I did not go around flirting with boys. I did not even know how. I would talk to them, but only those I knew through my brother, who had gone to the same high school two years ahead of me, or only a few in my class. Or only if they spoke to me first. I didn't even have a boyfriend.

I still question why she called me that when she did not really know me. What image did I project? I had a reputation at school for being shy and quiet. All the teachers knew that. Most of my classmates knew that.

I will never know the answer.

I still struggle with issues of low self-esteem and self-confidence. I have days where I cannot stand to look at my own reflection.

I remember saying something to this effect to someone when I was in my 30s.

"You're too old to be thinking that way," was pretty much the reply.

I still wonder what my age has to do with it. Is there a certain point where we are not supposed to care about what other people think of us? I would like to think that at the end of it all, none of it really matters.

For most of the people who passed by in my life, I would

probably be just a blip on the radar. They would have little idea that the things they said to me, added together, would have such an impact. This is my reality.

If I should not care so much about what people think about how I look, why do we have women being photographed in heavy make-up? Why have make-up at all? If appearance matters so little, it begs the question. Why are there so many young girls wearing clothing or cosmetics designed to hide who they really are?

Let's face it. The media sells an image that, to most of us with at least a modicum of common sense, is fake. Yet there are various illnesses that, in many respects, are the direct result of being sold these fake images. Depression, poor self-esteem, anorexia nervosa, bulimia and dozens of other related problems can be traced back to this.

This is not meant to be an indictment of the modelling industry, or Hollywood. This is more a pointing out of the double standard that exists when people say: "you shouldn't care so much about what people think of you". The truth is we all care. Maybe too much.

This is also not to say that my self-esteem issues are the direct cause of my illness. I have my theories on how my illness developed, and there are several factors. My problems with my self-image are just one small part of it.

The hardest thing that I still need to get over is the idea that people come and go in my life. I have people who I once considered friends, but I am lucky now if I hear from them once a year. It is a tough one and sometimes gives rise to negative thoughts and feelings that maybe they were never really friends and only tolerated me.

No one said being around someone who has depression is easy. Goodness knows, a person in a depressive mood can suck the energy out of a room. In my experience, I have always been fairly reluctant to take part in things, mostly because my natural reserve stops me from speaking up, thinking I do not have anything relevant to add to the discussion.

Another reason is the fear that I will say something wrong. I tend to be ultra-sensitive to certain things and react badly when someone says something that I am sensitive about. It is like something a friend described to me. She called it verbal diarrhoea.

I am not trying to be negative when I say that I have become resigned to the fact that some people are just not meant to find that one person, that one great love. I have not gone on a date in years. In many ways, I am too scared to try. I have had one real relationship and the one thing I remember thinking the whole time we were going out was: Why? What do you see in me that makes you want to be with me?

Part of it comes down to that image I have of myself that I am not worthy of such a relationship. So, I have tended to hide away.

It is also why I feel sometimes I can never have a real relationship with other members of my family. I tend to be too critical of their faults, although I am ten times more critical of myself. I would rather hide away or stay away from family gatherings for fear I will say something that comes out wrong and end up hurting someone or being an embarrassment to them. They do not really understand why I am the way I am and will probably never understand.

There is yet another part of me that still feels that I was to blame for the problems in my immediate family. As if my birth created a jinx that they never really could get rid of. It sounds ridiculous, but I did often wonder if my parents would have been better off if I had never been born.

I often think: what if my parents had divorced? Would I have lived with my mum, in which case my life would probably have changed for the better, or would I have ended up going with my dad and never have achieved anything I did achieve?

Hindsight is 20-20, of course, and I do feel that had my

mother not been able to win the arguments with my father over my desire for an education and my desire to move away from home, I would not have done half the things I did. He was that repressive.

I still have to fight these thoughts, especially on my low days. I have more good days than bad now, although I still get stressed out sometimes. Financial struggles are a big part of that. Unfortunately, the desire to win Lotto isn't enough to make it a reality.

In many ways, while I am doing okay, I am still struggling to overcome the root cause of my depression, and I still have days where I want to scream. As much as I would like to think something like having a huge financial windfall would make all my problems go away, there is no magic pill.

Doctors are making breakthroughs all the time and have learnt much about mental illness, yet it is the one area where they still have a long way to go. The best anyone with this illness can hope for is to manage it.

Some might ask: why can't you just let all this go? Why can't you just get over it? For the same reason someone with everything to live for might decide suicide is the only way out. Because sometimes the voices we have inside us that tell us we're not good enough can overwhelm us to the point that nothing else we tell ourselves can drown out those voices.

It is a sad fact that no one can really truly understand what it is like for someone going through depression; even someone who has depression themselves. It is not a lack of empathy, and this is not a failing in itself; no one can walk a mile in another person's shoes. It is just not possible.

My hope is that by raising awareness through campaigns, telling stories like mine and the others in this book, we can enlighten others and change the way they view such illnesses.

Chapter Two: The Beginning

Part of learning to manage my illness was seeing those around me from a different perspective. To understand why certain people in my life behaved the way they did, I had to look at who they were and where they came from.

I grew up in a small city near the bottom of the North Island of New Zealand, about two hours' drive from the capital city. Palmerston North was not a bad place to grow up in. I have lived elsewhere, and, contrary to some observations, it is not as boring a place as one would think.

The year I was born, 1971, was at the tail end of the flower power generation. The Vietnam War was still raging and would not officially end with American withdrawal for another four years. Back in New Zealand, the average Kiwi was relatively unaffected by what was going on in South-East Asia. Our troops were pulled out of the conflict that year, as were Australia's.

That year saw conflicts between India and Pakistan, the opening of Disney World in Florida and China was admitted to the United Nations. It saw the debut of the Nasdaq stock market index, a devastating earthquake in Peru and the IRA bombed the Post Office tower in London. Idi Amin began his dictatorship with the taking over of Uganda and notorious killer Charles Manson, along with three of his followers, was sentenced. He would receive the death penalty but managed to escape execution due to a technicality. He died in 2017.

In popular culture, *Love Story* with Ryan O'Neal and Ali McGraw was one of the top movies, Jim Morrison of The Doors was found dead, and *The Partridge Family* was a high-rating TV show.

In New Zealand, Keith Holyoake was Prime Minister, and the National Party was in power.

Arthur Allan Thomas was found guilty of the murders of Harvey and Jeannette Crewe. He would eventually receive a pardon. Famed opera singer Kiri Te Kanawa made her debut in Covent Garden. There were anti-Vietnam protests in Queen Street, Auckland in May, Manapouri power station was completed, and scheduled steam-hauled service on New Zealand Railways came to an end.

My father, David, was born the year war was declared in Europe. It was summer in the southern hemisphere. Hitler was already starting his rampage across Europe and would invade Poland later that year. It was a tough time with many people still suffering from the effects of the Great Depression.

My paternal grandparents, Eileen and Leslie were New Zealand born and bred. Both were first generation Kiwis, their families having come to the country in the late 19th century.

My most vivid memories of my grandfather were of a rather taciturn man. I would not like to say I was afraid of him, but I barely remember any affection from him. My grandmother worried about me a lot. I think she knew early on that I had mental health issues, although this was a subject rarely discussed in the '80s when I was a teenager.

Grandad joined the Air Force and was part of the Home Guard during the war. My grandmother once told me he did a lot of his training at what is now Arena Manawatu in Palmerston North, not far from where I grew up. They lived in Pukerua Bay in those early years, and Grandad worked in Wellington.

Dad spent much of his childhood and early teen years on farms. His parents had a farm in Eketahuna in the Wairarapa in the late 1940s until about 1951. He would often tell stories of going out on cold mornings in Eketahuna and standing with his feet in a still-steaming cowpat.

After they left Eketahuna, they had a farm at Puhipuhi, a tiny settlement north of Hikurangi. When I was a child, my father took us to the area, and my grandmother showed us an old mine not far from where the farm used to be. My only memory is of the land being overgrown and covered in gorse.

My father's secondary school education consisted of correspondence. I assume this was because Puhipuhi was too far for a school bus to travel in the 1950s. He completed two years of this education and did not progress to what I knew as fifth-form level (year 11 today).

He went on to join the Air Force, but there is some confusion around how he joined. The story I heard was that he begged his parents to give him permission to join up even though he was a minor. Another story I heard was that my grandmother pushed him into it. Whatever it was, he did not last long in the Air Force. He did not have the maths skills to allow him to train as a pilot, and he took lessons to gain his private pilot's licence. At least, that was the story he told me. I have learnt to take a lot of the things he told me with a grain of salt.

My mother was born as Jennifer Carroll. Her parents were both New Zealand-born, but their families came from both Europe, Ireland, and the UK, via Australia in some cases. My great-grandfather was awarded a medal for service in World War I, following an incident in which he saved fellow soldiers (This was described in a book on medals given to servicemen in World War I).

My grandparents lived in a little village called Tinui, near Masterton, when my mother was born at the very end of 1946. World War II had ended, and she became part of the 'baby-boomer' generation.

She has happy memories of Tinui although she did not get along well with her older sister, nor with her mother. She has told of being forced to babysit her little sister when she was not more than a child herself, and of punishments where her mother would smack her children with the jug cord (something that would be considered physical abuse nowadays).

She has fond memories of her father, a jovial man, who was considered a bit of a joker, as was his father.

I can still remember as a six-year-old meeting my great-grandfather at the War Veterans' Home in Levin. I was so shy that I tried to hide behind my mother rather than talk to him, but he soon had me giggling. He died a year later and was the only great-grandparent I ever met. The rest passed away before I was born.

My grandparents always seemed to bicker, but while my grandmother was considered something of a harridan, my grandfather gave as good as he got. He would tease her endlessly. Their bickering could escalate into full-on arguments. When I was in my first year at university, my grandmother broke her leg (it may have been her ankle or her knee). I went to stay with them for a few days to help out and witnessed an argument between them. They were together almost 60 years, so it is unsurprising there would be a few fights.

Nana and Grandad moved around a lot. My mother once calculated they moved house about 40 or more times (in different towns each time) during their marriage. My grandfather was a mechanic, a career my mother once considered herself, but sadly in the 1960s, this was not possible. I wonder sometimes if their bickering and the moving reflected more than just a general unhappiness in my grandmother.

As a teenager, my mother attended Otaki College, and she did well in school, but she only completed third and fourth form. She was badly injured in an accident on her bicycle shortly before she turned 15 and did not go back to school the next term. Instead, she began working full-time.

She worked for a lawyer's office at one point during the 1960s. During that same period, her parents moved to Feilding. Mum once told me that she was forced to give up her job at the lawyer, but she eventually took on a job Hopwoods in Main Street, Palmerston North, as secretary-to-the-buyer. This store would, many years later, become a Mitre 10. My father was working as a storeman-driver there.

Dad used to joke that my mother was the one who chased him, because she would go out to where he was working to talk to him. Several months later, they married in a registry office.

To say my grandparents were not happy was something of an understatement. They felt that my parents had not known each other long enough. I later felt that my grandmother looked down on my father for various reasons, least of which, is that he was 'the wrong class'.

I can remember my parents always complaining that my grandmother never visited, unless she was 'on her way' to somewhere else. The grandparents would stop in long enough for lunch but would soon be on the road again.

My grandmother could be very critical, yet, at the same time, I felt unfairly singled out by her. She would buy things for me but wouldn't do the same for my brother. Her reasoning was that he was working, yet, I was working too, so it made little sense.

Most of her grandchildren, up until my teens, were boys. I had one female cousin, older than me, who was adopted, but my theory was that I was singled out because I was her biological grand-daughter. I cannot say for sure if my cousin received the same kind of attention. I have a younger female cousin who was born when I was in my teens. However, I cannot say for sure whether she received the same kind of attention I did.

Chapter Three: Childhood

My family was not rich. When I was born, up until I was five years old, we lived in a two-storey unit in a poor area of the city; Croydon Avenue, in Takaro. It would later become known for its gang activity and I have since learnt this began to occur around the same time we lived there.

The unit we lived in was a state house. In the 1930s, as a way of helping families affected by the Great Depression, the new Labour Government developed a scheme to build homes for low-income families.

According to Housing New Zealand, the Government corporation that administered all state-owned housing, the unit was built in the 1960s. My mother recalls when she and my father first moved in, the place was crawling with fleas. My brother was only a few months old at that time, and there was no way she would put him down on a floor that was basically black with the pests. The kitchen had not fared any better. The maintenance hadn't been kept up very well.

That place gave my mother a few bad moments. When I was a baby and learning to crawl, my father was supposed to have been watching me, but I somehow managed to elude him and fell down the stairs. My brother also gave my mother a fright one day when she was out in the garden, only to look up and see him standing at an open window on the upper floor. She often says she had never run so fast in her life.

The room that became my bedroom was so small I often felt claustrophobic. I was terrified of the dark and had nightmares.

When I was five, we moved into another state house in Robinson Crescent, Westbrook. This one was a brand-new house in a new suburb. The suburb was so new, no-one knew where it was and we'd explain it was next to Highbury, which, even then, did not have the best reputation. The house was brick with wooden frames and aluminium joinery. We were its first tenants. That three-bedroom house would be our home for the next 18 years.

Being a new suburb, there was still much development going on. New families moved in. Some bought the new homes while others, like my parents, were paying an extra amount in the hope of saving up a deposit so they could buy the house.

The house had a number of faults. The wood used for the framing was green and over the years it shrunk. The back door opened the wrong way, blocking off the doorway to the laundry. The windows often had very bad condensation in the winter, causing water to drip down, onto the wallpaper. The shower leaked and rotted the chipboard flooring underneath, which crept through into the room I was supposed to have. I was a rather sickly child, prone to bronchial infections every winter. My brother ended up moving into that room for a while.

In the dining room, we had huge windows on three sides. Palmy is notorious for its equinoctial winds which tend to blow for months at a time, and these windows had a lot of give in them. Whether the aluminium joinery had been badly constructed is hard to say, but my father would often comment that he feared the windows would smash, or worse. He would often put his hand on the glass in those high winds and feel the wind pushing the glass inward.

Next door to our house was a paddock. We had heard it was

owned by the Board of Education, and there was a proposal to build a school there. Instead, sometime after my parents moved out, they extended the park the land backed onto.

That paddock brought with it rats and mice, as well as various creepy-crawlies. I was always rather fearful and had phobias. My father didn't help.

I remember one incident when I was older. He had been out collecting snails in the garden and had an ice-cream container full of them. I was loading washing into the machine when he came in, standing in the doorway of the laundry, with the container full of snails. I hated them and still do. He effectively trapped me in that laundry with that container in his hands, even knowing I had a phobia. To him, it was a huge joke, but I was practically screaming.

Despite the faults, I had a lot of good memories of that house. I had a pet – a cat named Chippy. As much as my father tried to stop me, I ran around, playing games with the neighbour's kids, climbed trees and explored the banks of the Mangaone Stream.

My brother, who was two years older, and I, would often visit his then-best friend to play with his Star Wars action figures. He had a huge collection of figures from the movies, and we were early fans.

I had a fairly happy childhood. I would like to say I had no troubles at all, but sadly that is not the case.

I don't recall ever attending Playcentre or kindergarten. I may have gone once or twice, but my first days in formal education were at Takaro School. I was already somewhat advanced for my age in reading. I was able to read my brother's readers at three.

I have very few memories of Takaro. Most of them were not happy memories. On my fifth birthday, I had been given my first school bag. It was a neon orange bag, which was apparently the fashion in the mid-70s. My mother also made sure I had my own, special lunchbox with a Holly Hobbie sticker on it. That lunchbox did not last long. Theft was rife at Takaro.

Around the time we moved from Takaro to Westbrook, I had an accident at the school. I can barely recall what happened other than the fact I fell from the top of a fort in the playground. The fall was probably only two or three metres, but to a child my size, it was a serious fall. I was told later that the teacher made me get up and walk to the office, despite possible injuries to my back. My parents were angry at how I was treated, and I spent a few days at home. My mother was working part-time then, doing home help, and my mornings were spent at a neighbour's.

We transferred to Highbury School (which many years later was renamed Somerset School). I had five, mostly happy, years at that school although there were a few moments that would go on to shape my own feelings about my self-image. I participated in a few things, including being a student librarian, helping out on the crossing patrol and playing netball.

At five, I was yet to start wearing glasses. My mother recalls that I had a lazy eye and I was made to wear a patch over my left eye to get the right eye to work properly, although I don't have any memory of this.

I do remember that I began to have problems with my teeth. I have no idea why my teeth became so prominent. My mother had the same problem as a child, so perhaps it was genetic. Her own theory was that, as a toddler, I would suck on the corners of a small blanket, or suck my thumb. My parents could not afford the treatment I would need to straighten my teeth and there was no help from the government. It was considered cosmetic, yet I have had various problems caused by an overbite.

I have a photo, taken of me at five, my first one at Highbury School. My lips are pressed together in a sort of grimace, and I refused to smile widely, showing my teeth. It seems rather telling that at five years old, I was already sufficiently aware of self-image that I refused to smile properly in that photo.

When I was eight, a test at school revealed I had trouble seeing the words on the blackboard. My parents took me to an optician, and I began wearing glasses. Those glasses were and have always been the bane of my life.

I barely recall how many children had glasses in those days, so it was something of a novelty. It wasn't long before I was nicknamed 'four eyes'. My parents tried to tell me to ignore it, or laugh it off by saying: "Four eyes are better than two", but it was a very painful experience in many ways.

I was already beginning to have poor self-esteem issues. Being a 'poor kid', living in a state house, was a major issue. I had few friends, being too shy to form lasting friendships. I remember there was one boy who made fun of me for my shyness. Despite being in one of the top groups academically in primary school, I barely participated in class discussions.

That in itself was an issue that would crop up now and again. As shy as I was, being put in one of the top groups didn't make things any easier for me. While I never considered it showing off, I had a well-developed vocabulary and tended to use 'big words', yet other children would see me as showing off.

I would not like to say I was resented for it but there was a rather funny incident when I began Standard Two - I think this is about Year Four - where I do wonder if there was some kind of rivalry that I was previously unaware of. I had always been a good speller and that year I started off at a higher level of spelling than a boy who was a little older than me. I would later develop a sort of crush on the boy, although I'm embarrassed to admit it now. When he discovered I had surpassed him in spelling, he was stunned. "Why are you above me?" was pretty much his response.

I would often hang around with the kids who were below my level academically. While they did not make fun of me, per se, it always felt like I was 'tolerated' in a sense. I had few friends at school and felt like I did not fit in with the smart kids, or any of the other groups really.

Another issue was my last name. That became the subject of much teasing as well. World War III was one of the phrases used to tease me.

When I was about nine or ten, a young boy, probably around my age, began taunting me. He lived not far from us in a cul-de-sac. The boy would cycle past me, calling out names and generally being very rude. I had no idea who this boy was or why he would do such a thing. My brother, having heard this, chased after the boy and demanded to know why he was saying such things to me. The boy's excuse was that I had done the same thing to him. I barely had the confidence to open my mouth, let alone say anything cruel to anyone. It is just not in me to be that cruel. My brother told the boy off and made it perfectly clear I would never tease someone.

It was one of the few times I actually saw my brother defend me in such a way, despite the fact we often fought.

Primary school was not all bad. There were times when, looking back, I realise a couple of the boys did like me – it seems odd now that we place so much importance on social relationships and whether we're liked in a 'more than friends' way, but it was partly due to the era I grew up in. While feminism had been around about a decade, I was yet to learn about such things.

We had a graduation, of sorts, when we moved from primary level to intermediate - some people would call that middle school now. For this graduation, we were sent to the school hall and made to learn different dances for the Standard Four Social. My brother had had to do the same thing two years earlier, so I understood. His dance included some moves from the movie *Saturday Night Fever*. Disco was very popular then.

I recall very clearly a red dress with small flowers that was one of my favourite dresses to wear to school. I wasn't necessarily a 'girly-girl' but I was no tomboy either. That dress did earn me a few compliments from some of the boys in my year.

As I grew, however, things changed. Compliments became few and far between.

I moved on to Intermediate after Standard Four and found a rather different world. For one thing, we had to wear a school uniform. This may still be an ongoing argument among many schools here in New Zealand - that wearing a uniform prevents children being set apart from others due to their parents' socio-economic status. Even at the age of ten, it was obvious that some children were teased because of this.

While some of the kids from my old school transferred over, we were separated into different classrooms and I had to find new groups of children to hang around with. Not that I was very social. I would play on the playground, but I didn't have that many friends I could confide in.

My world view began to change in the two years I was at that school. For instance, we were studying a unit on prejudice. I was so sheltered that racism and prejudice didn't really affect me. Looking back, I would assume it went on, but I most likely never noticed it.

Our teacher chose to try an experiment with us. We were separated into groups: for instance, those with brown eyes and those with blue eyes. For half the day, those with blue eyes were considered 'superior' to everyone else, and we were allowed to make fun of the other group. The next half we swapped it around. I do not think anything truly hurtful was ever said, but I may be wrong on this point.

The teacher asked us to write our observations and feelings on a piece of paper and hand it in. We were not to give our names. She read out some of the notes. One in particular stood out, implying that the student had always felt 'inferior'. In many ways, I considered the experiment to have been a failure. I know my teacher's heart broke when she read out that statement. I could hear it in her tone.

I suppose in a way I began to face my own kind of prejudice. The older I grew, the more my 'differences' stood out.

When I was about twelve, I was called 'Bugs Bunny' - my teeth had become very prominent at this stage, and this boy, who could not have been older than 16, thought it would be a huge joke to call me that. My mother ripped into him. I was also called that by someone who was supposedly a friend of the family. He also received a telling off by my mother.

At that age, my body was still developing. I was small compared to others the same age, so anything like my teeth would have stuck out like a sore thumb.

Unfortunately, my parents could not afford braces. They could not get any help from the Government for them, because they were considered a 'cosmetic issue'. It was slightly different for when I had to get glasses. They were allowed to borrow an advance from what was then called Family Benefit to get those.

Chapter Four: Teenage Years

When I was young, my father was the one earning the wage, and it was not a lot of money. Back in the late '70s, it was about $140 a week, barely enough to support a family of four. Today's equivalent would be below minimum wage. There certainly were no savings, but that wasn't just because of the low wage.

Were we poor? I suppose by some standards we were. I prefer to think of us as low middle-class rather than working class. There was always a meal on the table, even if it was nothing fancy. My father had his faults, especially where money was concerned, but we never went without food. Luxuries were different.

I did not like admitting to the kids at my primary school that I lived in a state house. Being in that situation was considered not cool in those days, at least, by my perception. I suppose I had what one would call an inferiority complex. I thought my friends or fellow pupils were richer than me because their parents owned their own homes. I knew nothing of mortgages or market rents at five.

My father worked as a storeman at a small firm. Part of his job was to deliver groceries to various homes around Palmerston North. When I was off school, I would love to go with him in the van. Many of his customers would have little treats for me.

He chose to quit the job when I was 10. My mother told me that he did not tell her he was quitting, but just arrived home one day and told her he had done so. There had been no discussion.

He went on the unemployment benefit, and our financial situation became a lot worse. There were problems between my parents - not that I was aware of it at the time - revolving, of course, around money. We were a one-income family, and that didn't change.

My clothes were mostly either hand-me-downs or had been sewn by my mother, a skilled sewer. Children, unfortunately, can sometimes be the harshest of critics and they considered themselves superior if their clothes were bought for them. Never mind that the clothes my mother could make for me were often far better quality.

My mother was forced to go on the unemployment benefit when my father decided to leave and go to stay with his mother. I was in my first year at Intermediate. I believed, at the time, it was to look for a job so we could all move to Whangarei, where she lived.

My brother and I didn't make things easy for my parents. While we did play together as children, we also fought a lot. My mother had a hard job trying to cope with the two of us on her own.

She eventually found a job that paid better than what my father was paid in his old job, although that was the cause of some issues between them as well. I believe now he was jealous of that. Whether it was to do with her being a woman or something else is something I will never know.

When I was 11, I was in an accident. It was a rainy day, near the end of the school year. This I remember quite vividly as my brother, who was in college, was about to head off for his last day of term.

We had a dairy on the corner of our street. While there was car parking outside the shop, the drivers of delivery trucks had a habit of parking on the road outside the car park - basically double-parking, instead of around the corner where they didn't obstruct the view of drivers leaving the street.

I had just left home and was cycling to the end of the street. My glasses were fogging up, and my view was blocked by a truck double-parked. I didn't see the car coming until it was too late. I ended up hitting the side of the car and falling to the road.

I was lucky. I only ended up with cuts and bruises, and broken glasses, as well as a mild concussion. I was kept home that day and returned to school the next week. Of course, when I did return to school, I was asked to recount every detail of the accident for my fellow pupils. I was embarrassed by the whole thing and to this day still cringe when I think of it.

I was bullied through my teenage years. While the bullying seems mild in comparison to what goes on nowadays, any type of bullying or harassment is not okay.

When I was twelve, my nemesis was D****. She didn't seem particularly bright, and I suppose that was part of the reason she picked on me. I was known as a bit of a brain-box, even though I was too shy to volunteer answers in class. My teachers often despaired of ever being able to break me out of my shell.

I learnt sometime later that before my second year of intermediate, my teacher had arranged for me to join her class in that year. I believe she was trying to guide me in some way and help me break out of my shell.

In Intermediate, we were assigned manual classes. They may be called electives in other schools, but this was what I knew them by in my schooldays; not to mention the fact that they were compulsory. These classes were woodworking, metalwork, cooking and sewing. Each comprised of several weeks of these classes and all students did them in a rotation, i.e. cooking for eight weeks, sewing for eight weeks, etc.

I was in the cooking classroom one afternoon. My memory of why I was there isn't great - I think perhaps I was helping the teacher during lunch. D**** had earlier asked me in class if I wore a bra. A stupid thing to ask, and I told her that I didn't, as I hadn't developed yet. I was rather small and skinny for my age, and as I mentioned earlier, my vocabulary was fairly advanced. Some kids matured later than others.

She came in to the cooking classroom and yelled out: "Have you 'aveloped yet?" Yes, she did pronounce it that way. Wanting to get away from her, I left the classroom and ran to catch up with my friend. D**** caught up with me. I think she may have even dragged me back to the classroom.

"Don't you run away from me," she told me. She then slapped me.

I immediately went into shock. I had never been hit by anyone, other than my father's hidings, and to be hit by a fellow pupil was just not on. Of course, being the sensitive child that I was, I cried. Another girl, who apparently was also known as something of a bully, although she may have had a soft spot for me, asked me what happened. Had our teacher not come in, I am fairly certain there would have been a fight between the two girls.

I wasn't the only one D**** bullied. She did the same to a girl who became my best friend that year. Our teacher gave the excuse that D****'s home life was not ideal. I realised later that meant she was being hit by one of her parents, but to me, that never justified her behaviour toward me. I learnt a lesson that day about injustice.

Then in high school, there were three girls - one of whom I'd gone to primary school with, who decided I was also a target for their bullying. They stopped after a couple of years, but even at 16, I continued to be the target of bullies.

Then one day, I couldn't take it anymore. Another group of girls, who were two years behind me, seemed to make a sport of targeting me and a friend. I guess everyone has their breaking point, and this was mine.

One of those girls had been making fun of me because the

shoes I wore were not the style that most of the kids wore. My parents were not rich enough to buy those shoes as they were rather expensive. I also had a red jacket. This girl would call me "Little Red Riding Hood with her little brown shoes". I would try to tell my father or a teacher only for them to tell me to 'ignore it'. Ignoring it wasn't helping.

One lunch hour, my friend and I were sitting in our usual spot and the girls came along. They began throwing food at us, like orange peel. I had had it. I marched up to those girls and told them I was going to "kick their arses". They looked taken aback, their expressions like a 'deer in the headlights'. They clearly had never expected me to stand up for myself. They never went near us again. There was the occasional taunt if I happened to meet one of them in the corridor, but they never did it again.

School was, in many ways, my sanctuary. I loved learning and still do. While I participated very little in the social aspects of high school – I never went to school dances and was never asked out by boys, I did begin to come out of my shell a little. Even if I did turn bright red when called on in class. Part of me preferred to sit in the corner with my head down and not call attention to myself, which concerned many of my teachers.

I decided to leave school at the end of my sixth form year instead of staying one more year. My father did not discourage me from doing so. It is one of my few regrets. I sometimes wonder if I had stayed one more year whether I would have come out of my shell more.

If it is true that we are a product of our environment, then I can only surmise that the things that happened to me in my childhood were contributing factors to my illness. Certainly, my self-esteem issues stemmed from some of this.

Another contributing factor was my father.

Chapter Five: Dad

"Your brother was planned. You weren't."

The words might sound innocuous in themselves, but in the context of my father's behaviour toward me, it paints a completely different picture.

I was told my father was in the delivery room when I was born and was the first to hold me. He cried.

This was the early 1970s when hospitals were only just beginning to allow the fathers in delivery rooms to witness the actual birth. My brother was born in 1969 and Dad was sent to the waiting room, so he'd never actually seen my brother's birth.

I was in my late teens when this conversation took place. My father did not follow up with a rejoinder telling me I was wanted anyway. The background to what he said to me makes it sound much worse. When my mother got pregnant with me, my father accused her of cheating. That was not the case.

My mother did not find out about the conversation until after Dad had died from cancer. She was livid.

My relationship with my father had many ups and downs. When it came to punishment, he was the one who would dole that out.

I was a very introverted child, basically bottling up my emotions until it got to a point where I would explode. My father did not like my tantrums. His method of punishment was terrific hidings. He would always use his hand, but he was never gentle. They would be hard, painful smacks across the buttocks or the top of the thighs. Today, those smacks would be considered abusive in the context of child protection laws, but that kind of thing did not exist then.

I heard my dad crying after I had had one of these episodes, and been subsequently punished for it. I went to him and told him I loved him. He said: "I love you too, except when you're naughty."

Maybe I'm wrong, but a parent's love should be unconditional. Just because a child does something that is considered naughty, is that a reason to stop loving the child? Nothing I ever did deserved that.

I realise now that that simple statement has coloured all my relationships. I am always afraid I will not be loved if I behave badly.

When my mother began working full-time it was my father who took over the housekeeping duties. He would be there when I got home from school. He refused to get himself a part-time job, saying all the money he earned would go on rent. We were still paying rent to Housing Corporation and as Mum was working full-time, they charged market rent. Legally, they could not charge any more than that. His excuse didn't wash.

Dad was bored at home. He spent most of his time working out different formulas which he hoped would help him win money at the T.A.B. He was a gambler, forever spending money on horse racing. Had we had a casino in town, there was a good chance he would have spent all his time there.

Dad's gambling was a huge problem for us. Mum budgeted a certain amount each fortnight for housekeeping. The bills were always paid, and we had food on the table, but there was no money left over. Dad would spend it all on the races. Treats were a rarity. We never had money for decent holidays and would only go to stay with my grandmother in Whangarei. Up until the mid-'80s, both my parents smoked, but the good thing is we still didn't go without food. However, they still struggled to make ends meet. For all the money Dad spent on his gambling, we could have owned the house we lived in outright.

Anything they wanted, like a new dining room table, or a lawnmower, had to be bought on hire purchase. My father once begged my mother to buy a pool table on hire purchase, but the novelty soon wore off.

He was very hypocritical when it came to money. One day, when I was 24, I was talking to a friend on the phone about going to the movies. My father's reaction was typical.

"What do you want to do that for? You should stay home and save your money."

He could never save money himself, since he was gambling it all away.

I never dated in high school. It was not just that no one ever asked me. I never went anywhere. I was not allowed to get an after-school job. Dad was not happy when I managed to get a one-day job on a weekend doing stock-taking.

I once mentioned I would like to go out late at night. My father's answer was that he would rather I didn't, "because I'd have to get out of bed and come and get you."

Even as an adult, when I had my own transport, he was not happy about me going out with friends and wouldn't sleep until he knew I was home. That might sound normal for any parent, but in many ways, it was suffocating.

Imagine living with someone who constantly made you feel guilty for wanting a life; who never encouraged you in anything you wanted to do, who laughed at you whenever you tried to do something that wasn't the norm. I do not recall my father ever telling me I was pretty. In many ways, I think he was jealous of my academic ability. He questioned my desire to go to university, telling me I would never finish what I started. I proved him wrong. Twice. Although, by the second time, he had long passed.

I later learnt that for years, my mother had been running interference with my father. They would often fight over me because she wanted me to be able to get out and have friends. My father didn't want that. He was very possessive; of me, and my mother. He certainly did not like her going out. I remember one evening, my mother had a work function to go to. He did not want to let her go.

He had certain rules he lived by and seemed to expect the same from my mother and I. He never drank alcohol, although I have heard that he did when he was in the Airforce, just to be sociable. One year, my mother went to our neighbour's home to help her bake a Christmas cake. She came back tipsy – they had drunk more sherry than had gone in the batter. My father was furious with her.

Yet, where my brother was concerned, he could do anything he liked. When my brother announced he was going flatting with a friend, my father's reaction was to throw his hands up in the air and cry: "Hooray!" When I wanted to do the same thing, it was: "Are you sure you know what you're doing?" I was 23, older than others who had already gone flatting.

I firmly believe to this day that his negativity is what caused cancer to grow in his body. He used to say: "I'm not going to reach 65. In fact, I'm not even going to reach 60." He died at 59 years old from renal cell carcinoma (kidney cancer).

Some years ago, before my father died, I mentioned some of the things he did to a woman who was a counsellor.

"That's abuse," she said.

At the time, I probably was not sufficiently self-aware to realise what she really meant. I have also read that most people who have experienced this type of abuse do not know they are being abused and can only recognise it when they are removed from it. I do not know how true this is and I certainly cannot speak for someone who has experienced physical abuse. I only know that it is true for me. I know now, looking back, that what he did to me was emotional abuse. I am not saying it was worse than physical abuse, but I do believe they are both equally as bad.

We would have our share of arguments. When I first went to university, I would talk to him about things I had learnt there. One particular time, we began arguing about a certain topic that had a lot to do with some of New Zealand's cultural history. No matter what proof I offered that Dad's view of historical events was wrong, he was convinced he was right.

This is not to say that I do not have some good memories of my father. A huge family joke was that he would often complain when someone in a car passed with their stereo blaring. Yet when certain songs came on the radio, especially in his own car, up would go the volume.

We both loved the black comedy M*A*S*H, about American doctors in a mobile army surgical hospital in the Korean War. No other show in my memory combined such black humour and pathos in the same episodic format.

It was one of those shows that taught me that when it comes to depression, sometimes having a sense of humour and learning to use it, even at what might seem to others to be inappropriate times, was the only way to help me get through the worst of it.

Dad had a laugh that could send someone into hysterics. The laugh was very similar to Alan Alda's - the actor who played Hawkeye in M*A*S*H. There was one particular episode that had us both in hysterics. The episode involved a rash of thefts around the camp. The C.O. Henry Blake, played by McLean Stevenson, was searching Hawkeye's tent for some of the items. The stove was used to heat the tent, otherwise known as The Swamp. In removing the chimney, Henry ended up with soot all over his face and Hawkeye was practically rolling on his bunk, laughing hysterically.

Dad would be laughing so hard I wouldn't be able to control my own laughter and have to leave the room. We had seen that episode many times but it never failed to make him laugh.

Since I have been working with a counsellor, I have begun to see my father from a different perspective. My paternal great-grandfather died when my grandfather was about three-years-old. My great-grandmother remarried five years later. So, it is not a huge stretch to assume that my grandfather missed out on having a male role model in the most formative years of his childhood.

Like most children who grew up during the war and post-war years, it would have been difficult for my father to have turned to his father for advice. The war was tough on everyone, and that would have caused problems in a lot of families. It is not difficult to believe that even though my grandfather didn't go overseas, his experience would have made him less likely to form any close bond with my father.

At that time, as isolated as New Zealand was, the war came very close to our shores. That would have been frightening for everyone concerned, regardless of whether they were serving in the armed forces. My grandmother once told me that, while still living in Pukerua Bay, they had a bag packed in case they needed to 'head for the hills'.

It is more than likely that many of the men who served both at home and abroad returned from their experience with some form of post-traumatic stress. Looking back, I can recall times when my grandfather appeared a little closed-off.

My maternal grandfather never talked about his experience in the war either, and he did go overseas.

Couple that with growing up in isolation, never being given the opportunity for an education, I can now see that my father's behaviour towards me was born out of his own bitterness about what he saw as his failures. Failure to achieve his dreams, failure to give his family security. He came from a generation that taught him the man was the breadwinner, and seeing my mother earning more money than he could ever have earned in his own work must have been another blow to his ego.

I firmly believe that Dad had a mental illness. I have read

theories that suggest being raised by someone with a mental illness can make a child more susceptible to it. His was never diagnosed. I suspect he refused to acknowledge it.

Seeing him from that perspective has allowed me to get to a point where I can forgive most of what he did. There are some things which still hurt, mostly because I do not think I can ever come to some understanding of why he did the things he did. At least now I can think of him with if not fondness, at least a sense of nostalgia, and without pain or anger.

Chapter Six: Diagnosis

I was 17 when my doctor diagnosed me with depression. Looking back, I am fairly certain that the symptoms began much earlier, but I lacked the knowledge to understand why I was feeling the way I did at that time.

One telling episode was when, during a school assembly a year before, the whole school was told that a student had died from brain cancer. Many of us broke down. Looking back, I believe now that this was an early symptom of my depression My reaction was out of proportion as I didn't even know the student although I had learnt that my brother's former best friend had been diagnosed with a brain tumour some years earlier.

Because of this issue, I was sent to relaxation sessions with a teacher once a week.

Not long after I left school, I would meet a friend in town for lunch, and we would spend a few hours together. I had difficulty getting a job, which probably contributed to my low self-esteem. My friend was also unemployed at the time.

We had met through school. She was as shy as I was and in many ways was as much an outsider among our classmates as I was. She had also been bullied by the same girls who used to do it to me.

We would often meet during lunch break, just sitting and

talking about all the usual teenage angst. We both decided to leave school the same year.

One particular day we had been out window shopping and had lunch at the local fast-food restaurant. We had gone to the local department store and were heading upstairs on the escalator when I began feeling nauseated. She was on the step above me.

"Go! Go! Go!" I urged. We both ran to the ladies' bathroom, where I promptly threw up in one of the sinks. Eventually, someone alerted staff, and they called my father to come and get me.

I have no idea if this was an episode of real sickness or if it was psychosomatic. What I do remember is that this episode led to more episodes of vomiting - enough that my parents became concerned that I was actually physically ill.

I would have episodes of cold sweats, terrible nausea, and I would hyperventilate, feeling like I had a huge weight on my chest. Some years later, I identified these as anxiety attacks. I almost became a shut-in, barely able to function and not wanting to go anywhere. These are classic symptoms of anxiety attacks, although they are not the same for everyone.

My doctor told me the symptoms were 'psychosomatic'.

I was taken aback. Psychosomatic, to me at that point, meant 'crazy'. Was I about to be locked up in the mental ward?

I was not a big fan of the doctor. There were many times I wondered if he considered me to be a hypochondriac. I had been going to the same GP since I was six. and I did not have a great rapport with him. I was forever going to him for migraines and various mystery ailments. I was not a well child, although I often wonder whether it was because my father, being over-protective as he was, might have been thinking the worst.

I did not know very much about mental illness at seventeen. I was very sheltered and often felt suffocated by my father's sense of over-protectiveness. I was naïve and extremely immature.

It makes me wonder now if something he did was the catalyst,

like a subtle nudging every now and again forcing me to turn inward. To repress my innermost desires and never fight for what I wanted, which manifested into a physical symptom.

So, all these circumstances added up to the beginning of my struggles. My knowledge of my illness and the whys and wherefores are based on years of self-analysis, of trying to understand where it had all come from.

Chapter Seven: Battles

The next few years were a struggle. I spent those four years barely able to function, although I did manage to get a summer job fruit-picking one year, which led to a frightening (for me) experience when a guy I didn't even know kissed me.

We had stopped for lunch and I was sitting beside the rows of strawberries. The young man sat next to me. He grabbed my bag and looked as if he was going to go through it. To stop him, I grabbed an apple from the bag and gave it to him. His next action was to kiss me. "I love you," he said.

I had no experience of men at this point, and this set off further issues with anxiety.

I decided to do a course in administration, hoping it would lead to a job. This was a scheme provided by the government where we could still receive the unemployment benefit and they would pay all costs involved with the course.

Admittedly the course did boost my confidence and give me some much-needed life skills, but on my first day, I had a massive anxiety attack. I had been seeing a counsellor and, knowing I was having the attack, went straight around to see him. He was not able to see me but the receptionist, a very kind woman, helped me calm down. She placed a call to the tutor and told her what I was going through.

I eventually did go to the course, which was based at what

was then Manawatu Polytechnic at a very lovely part of Palmerston North in Centennial Drive. The tutor persuaded me to give it a try and took me down to the classroom. I sat in on the first day of orientation and eventually calmed down enough to begin to enjoy it. Once I got through that first day, I was able to complete the three-month course, resulting in further qualifications in typing.

A year or so later, the government introduced a scheme which, at the time, was the best thing that could have ever happened to me. While I do have some regrets over it, I would never have been able to do what I did without it. The year was 1991, and the government had announced the introduction of the Student Loan Scheme. With it, I would be able to go to university – something I had always dreamed of doing, but since there was no possible way to save the money for a three-year degree, I had no other way of going.

Getting to university was not quite that easy. I had to apply for special admission as I had not completed seventh form. The admission requirements were that I had to be aged 20 or over (I would be 21 that year) and have Sixth Form Certificate, which I had.

In terms of getting the loan, I had to prove my parents had no money and no means of paying for my tuition. Due to some changes in how the government saw people my age, I could not apply for things like the Student Allowance without my parents' consent, because I was under 25. Apparently, they considered that anyone under 25 was not independent, yet I had basically been independent for years, even though I was still living with my parents.

So, in February of 1992, I enrolled at university. My first class was terrifying. I remember having an anxiety attack, and I had deliberately not eaten breakfast before I left home, thinking if I didn't eat, there would be less chance of me throwing up. This was a constant pattern where I would skip a meal in case I had an attack. My theory was that if there were nothing in my stomach, there would be nothing to throw up. It didn't stop the nausea, but it helped.

I had to tell myself that I was doing this for my benefit. If I didn't, I would prove my father right that I would never finish what I start. Getting the nerve to actually enter that lecture theatre was a struggle, but I did it.

Over the three years of my studies, I had many struggles, but I also had many wonderful moments.

I discovered the university had a campus newspaper. Eager to learn more about journalism, I asked about it and talked to the co-ordinator. He liked my enthusiasm and suggested I come to the volunteers' meeting. I joined the newspaper, but I wasn't confident enough to tackle a big story. Tim, the co-ordinator, was nice enough to help me build that confidence by giving me news briefs to work on. I also met the then editor, Richard, who was always nice to me. I was told he was a bit of a flirt, but I would never have known if he was doing the same to me. I was very naïve in those days.

I began working at the newspaper on a column of newsbriefs. One day, I had the opportunity to tackle what I felt was a 'real story'. I commented to Tim: "It's nice that I can write a real story." He seemed surprised by that.

His reply was: "I don't give a column to just anyone!" I loved that comment. I had never considered it a column but now that I think back on it, writing a news brief from an article, pulling out the gist of it without losing the impact, was actually something that took skill.

I thrived on university life. Maybe I didn't go to university events, like the toga parties they had during orientation week, but I felt I had found a place there, and the majority of my classmates were amazing people who didn't look down on me.

There were two professors in the English department whom I will credit with helping me gain more confidence in myself. Dick Corballis, who has since passed away, was the head of the English department and a lecturer who taught me much about English literature. The one thing I did take away from his classes was that no matter what we interpret from a poem or a piece of prose, there is never really a wrong or right answer. He was a wonderful teacher.

The second person is Robert Neale, a wonderful man who believed in my writing when I, at times, doubted myself. I will never forget his kindness and his encouragement.

My biggest struggle came when I had to participate in a quasi-debate for a history class. I would have to give one view and another student would give the opposite one. I was meant to go second, but I went to the professor (who was a visiting professor from Montana University) and told him how I was feeling. Bless that man for his understanding. It was the first time I had ever encountered someone in authority who didn't judge me for my illness, and even congratulated me for actually getting up there, despite my anxiety.

The one thing I did learn from that experience was that I could be open about it, although I still had to be cautious. Some people were not so understanding. While my personal knowledge of it was not that extensive, I was beginning to see that it was a lot more common than I realised.

I became friends with many of my fellow students. There was one student who once told me he admired me for my courage. For actually going to university despite my illness and actually succeeding. Maybe my grades weren't terrifically high, but I was still passing every class. I remember one thing he said to me:

"You don't realise the impact you have on other people."

They knew I struggled, with my family life, with my illness, although I doubt they really knew the full extent of it, or understood it, but they admired me for sticking with my studies.

When I was in my second year, I decided to try a modelling class to build my self-confidence. I certainly would never make it in the modelling industry, considering the girls have to be a minimum of about 1.7 metres tall and I'm shorter than that. The classes were held at a clothing shop in what was then Broadway Mall.

We were taught how to walk like models, how to comport ourselves like one and eventually we participated in fashion shows. The first one I did I got to wear my own clothes, but I was so nervous. The second one was a bridal show, held at the Convention Centre. It was fun, but in the second year of the course it was less fun and according to the teacher I was too stiff. I am not an actor, and I could not act relaxed to save my life. Some of the lessons did, however, manage to stick.

Some years later, when the photographer at the newspaper I worked at wanted to use up some of her colour film, I did some poses for her. The film was taken to be developed at the local store, since the paper didn't have the right equipment for developing colour photos, and the woman who checked the photos remarked on my poses and asked if I'd done any modelling. Which was rather flattering, I must say.

It is true that confidence shows and when I was at my most confident, it showed very well.

I met a girl at university who became my best friend. We would eventually go flatting together. Our friendship began to develop when we had to do a weekend workshop for a paper in drama. In the workshop, we were split into groups and told to rehearse five-minute plays, which would then be performed in front of the class at the end of the workshop. We had been placed in the same group.

She was almost three years younger than me, but we both felt a connection. We began spending a lot of time together, especially going to the movies. She was from a small town in Northland where they didn't have a multiplex cinema, and she went a little overboard with our multiplex - which had only been built a couple of years before - seeing movies almost every week.

She told me once I was difficult to get to know due to the

many walls I had around me. When she met my father, she began to understand. It helped that she was studying psychology, so she knew a little of what I was going through.

We decided to get a flat together in our third year. It wasn't easy. I certainly was not an easy person to live with. We had our share of fights, but we remained friends.

To this day, I still feel that one of the reasons I'm here is to teach others about mental illness. That while it may be a struggle, and it may be a burden, it's something we can all learn from.

Something else happened during those years at university that helped to shape my future.

Chapter Eight: Work and Life Changes

While I was studying for my degree in history and English, I signed up with Student Job Search.

I was hired for a temporary job working for a small organisation locally, just to do typing. It was only supposed to be one day, but I noticed the job required more than that. So I mentioned this to the manager and they hired me on a part-time basis, to work for a few hours every week. That job led to part-time work over the summer and would have most likely led to an offer of full-time work had I not been pursuing other avenues.

The women I worked with were absolutely lovely and meant a lot to me during that time. I was very moved when they both came to my father's funeral just a few years later. It meant more to me than they will ever know.

I found it laughingly ironic that I could not get a full-time job for four years, then went to university and scored a part-time job that gave me valuable experience. My third year at university, I also had another part-time job, typing student assignments. My skill base increased along with my experience as well as my self-confidence. I could actually hold down a job and study and be good at it.

After university, I applied to do a post-grad diploma in journalism in Auckland. By this time, my parents had moved further north, to Whangarei, ostensibly to look after my 84-year-old grandmother, who died that year. After I completed my studies, I moved in with them.

Sadly, I missed out on the post-grad course. I had applied for one at the local polytechnic, but that one was cancelled. I had also applied for one in Wellington but decided to withdraw my application.

Back on the unemployment benefit, I was sent as part of a 'work-for-the-dole' scheme to a school, eventually ending up being offered a part-time role there until my parents decided to return to my hometown. My grandmother passed away in December 1994 and they moved back to Palmy about October 1995.

Not wanting to stay on the unemployment benefit, I decided to return to university to complete a diploma. However, halfway through, my aunt told my mother about a job for a reporter at the *Levin Chronicle*. I applied, went for an interview, and got the job.

That job was hard in many ways, although I grew to love it. I'd always wanted to be a reporter, but I was still very naive and had difficulty finding my feet. It took several months for me to feel like I was swimming rather than sinking, and it appeared my boss felt the same way.

I found a small flat just a few minutes' walk away from the office, which was a huge advantage as we had early starts. We would start work at 7.30 in the morning. The Chronicle was a daily newspaper then, published six days a week. I was also the reporter for the Weekly News, a weekly community newspaper. On Fridays, we would start at 7am as we had to write stories for both the Friday and Saturday papers.

One funny incident sticks out in my mind. I was told in my first week the newspaper had a bar of sorts and on Fridays, after both the Friday and Saturday papers had been done, the staff would go up to the bar for drinks. My boss asked me if I drank, or smoked, to which I said no. He and the chief reporter looked at each other.

"Who is this woman?"

It's a well-known myth that journalists are heavy smokers and drinkers. That hasn't been the case for many years.

Some months into my tenure there, a man who was much older than I, kept asking me out for coffee. Still very naive when it came to men and relationships, and the fact that I didn't even know the man and certainly didn't like him, freaked me out. My boss was unsympathetic. "He's just a lonely man," he would say. I was placed in a horrible position where I felt I was being harassed and expected to just deal with it. Back then, we had no rules against sexual harassment.

I did not want to work with the man, who was essentially a freelancer. When the company announced they were opening up a new office in Paraparaumu, to expand the weekly newspaper, I was chosen to be its first reporter. The unfortunate problem was I now had to work with the same man, who had been contracted to supply photos for the paper.

I tried to keep things on a professional level, but he would complain to my boss about my attitude. I certainly was not trying to be a snob, or cold, but I was not going to be friendly either and have that misinterpreted. I was 26 and had little to no experience of relationships.

I enjoyed the responsibility of being the sole reporter for the Kapiti area, and even had the opportunity to take a few photos of my own. In many ways I still miss that job.

I left that job in January 1998, intending to move to Australia. It didn't work out that way. I moved back in with my parents in Palmerston North, and within six months, our lives changed completely.

My brother was living with us at the time, although he had enrolled in a film-making course at what used to be known as Avalon Studios in Lower Hutt. We moved to Levin, as my parents were hoping to find a place with cheaper rent. By the end of June, my father had been diagnosed with cancer.

I was at the hospital when Dad was diagnosed. The doctor told all of us, my father, my mother and I, that they had found a tumour on his kidney. My father started crying. I could tell from the look on his face that he was scared.

He was immediately booked for surgery so the kidney could be removed. A few days after he was discharged, the results came back. It was cancer. The doctors felt sure they'd got it all, but within days, Dad went downhill. He began vomiting blood and could barely stand up. He was readmitted to hospital around the beginning of August.

I was not working at this time. I had had knee surgery in June, and I was still recovering from that.

Driving back and forth from Levin to Palmerston North Hospital was gruelling. While Levin did have a hospital of sorts, it was only small and not equipped to handle cancer cases.

Levin is about half an hour's drive from Palmerston North. To get there, we either had to take a back road, or drive the Himatangi Straight, which, while a straight road, was also fairly open to high crosswinds. It could make driving a little treacherous.

Around the beginning of September, my father's sister flew down from Whangarei. While we had never had the easiest of relationships with her husband, he was the one who had told her to "get down there and see your brother".

My aunt stayed for the day and spent some time with my father. She was convinced he would be okay, yet there were several incidents that told me he was not going to make it.

It seems funny now, but at the time, it was alarming. My father appeared to regress, saying odd things that led my mother to believe he thought he was at a place he used to work at in his 20s. He would say odd things I couldn't understand. My best friend told me it sounded like he had multi-infarct dementia, which meant he'd had a series of small strokes. It was not an official diagnosis, but it did help explain the way he appeared to have lost a lot of his cognitive ability.

However, I believe there was more to it than that. On the Thursday, we met with his doctor who assured us Dad was doing fine. I tried pointing out a few things, but the doctor continued to give the impression he believed I didn't know anything. The next day, my father was sent for a full CT scan. My mother and I went home to Levin while he had the scan.

We had no sooner got home when we received a phone call. Mum picked up the phone and from the look on her face, I knew it was bad. My brother and I went down to the bedroom to listen in on the extension.

"Uh, I don't really like giving this kind of news over the phone," the doctor said.

"How long?" Mum asked, immediately knowing what the news was. "Weeks?"

"No."

"Days?" Her voice was breaking.

The cancer had spread. It was in his bones, his veins, and his brain.

I called a friend at the paper and asked her for the name of the Cancer Society volunteer co-ordinator. When I told the woman what was going on, she came around immediately. Bless her for her quick response. Without her, I think we would have all fallen apart.

It's amazing how, when you are faced with such a crisis, sometimes your brain can just kick into gear and do whatever has to be done. I remember thinking I had to be strong, that out of all of us, I was the one who couldn't fall apart, because my mother needed me.

Dad died three days later. I was numb; through the funeral service and for most of the next year. I would constantly dream that he was alive and that it had all been some horrible mistake. It took me four years to accept his death, and the only way I knew I had done so was because I had forgotten the anniversary.

Mum moved to Morrinsville a few weeks after Dad's death, renting a two-bedroom house her older sister owned. She regrets that, mostly because her sister could be very controlling, and it felt like she was taking over Mum's life. I went with her, planning to go to Australia a few weeks later.

I realise now that it was a mistake. No one who has gone through such a loss should think about making such major changes so quickly. So I came back from Australia and stayed in Morrinsville.

I was unemployed yet again and having difficulty getting a job. Then, in March of 1999, I sent a few letters to newspapers and was hired for a temporary job as a reporter for the paper in my hometown. Sadly, there was no further job offer. Part of that was my own fault. I didn't like what I was doing – I was given the role of agricultural reporter, something I had no knowledge of, and I just couldn't find my place. There may have been some personality clashes with some of the staff, and that didn't help my situation.

Around the anniversary of my father's death, my depression flared up again. It was due to a number of factors. Stress over trying to fit into a role I was not comfortable with, coupled with the thought that I would be once again looking for a job in a month's time, various health issues – not all of them my own, and restructuring within the company, it was little wonder it happened. I also believe that much of it was caused by the fact that I had never really grieved for my father's death. Despite our problems, I did love my father, and I missed him.

It was probably only a day or so before the anniversary when one of my colleagues saw me crying outside. I didn't tell them about the anniversary. Many of those I worked with did not appear to react well to my emotional state.

"We can see you're depressed," was all that they said. One person did suggest I see someone, and I did go to see a psychologist at the hospital.

My depression would flare up again a year later and

continue to do so for the next few years. It would become almost a roller-coaster of emotional turbulence.

I do not know if my depression was the reason I was not invited to stay on at my hometown newspaper, or whether this was one of the reasons I have never been successful in getting a role as a reporter since I left the newspaper in Auckland some years later. I did feel at the time that many people were not understanding of my situation.

Once again unemployed, I begged for a job with the same people I had once done strawberry picking for. They now had a business selling cut flowers to overseas buyers. It was not a job I liked, and there were times when I had clashes with one of the owners. Put it this way: I had a bad migraine that lasted two days. Her response was: "It's just a headache!" She saw no reason why I could not work, yet had no idea just how debilitating that migraine was.

A few months later, I applied for a job at a company which was opening a branch in my hometown, but even this was not to last. The company, while it was a government department, was losing money. A few months after I joined, I received a phone call from my team leader.

"Don't come into work tonight." The same message was given to everyone. We were told not to talk to the media. We soon found out why. The company had been placed into receivership. We returned to work the next shift not knowing if we would still have our jobs or what was going to happen.

It became a waiting game as we heard all kinds of rumours. Eventually, the company was sold, and work carried on as normal. However, the work for our branch dried up. We would spend half our time either reading or a small group would end up playing 'hackysack', a game I refused to take part in.

Fed up, I decided to hand in my resignation and left, a month before they decided to close down the branch. I moved to Hamilton, where my mother was living, and spent a few weeks on the unemployment benefit before getting a temporary role at a call centre. Still intent on further study, it worked as a stopgap until February the next year when I was able to join the degree programme for a Bachelor of Communication Studies at AUT in Auckland. I would not move from the city for 12 years.

After three years of study, I covered one reporter at a community newspaper when she went on a short leave of absence. That led to a fulltime job as a reporter for the Western Leader, another community newspaper in Henderson, Auckland. While I quickly found my feet, I made a lot of mistakes. It did not help that I was made fun of constantly by one person at this company. In front of my colleagues. It amounted to nothing short of harassment and began to erode my self-esteem. I was getting stressed and ended up on 'report' several times. I did not have the nerve to call out this person on their harassment and tell them they were the chief cause of my stress.

Credit where credit was due, I was allowed time out to seek help for my stress. This may have been ordered by head office, although I will never know. I was never able to confront the bully with the actual reason why my mental health once again began to go downhill.

My depression began to rear its ugly head by this stage. Two and a half years later, I left the paper, again intending to travel, but again it didn't work out. I found myself unemployed yet again, a stressful time in itself. I was unable to pay my bills and was humiliated when I had to go for a Nil Asset Procedure. This is one step short of bankruptcy for those who are unable to pay their debts. I also lost my car.

It was at this point that I began writing fanfiction for a TV show. Why this particular show is hard to say. There were a lot of faults in the writing and some of the episodes could have been done better, so perhaps that was the thing that prompted me to write these stories. There was something about it that kept me watching, despite all the faults.

I wrote my first fanfiction story a little over two years before the show came to the end of its ten-year run and posted it to an online community. Through that story, I made one friend, who lives in the Netherlands. Having lived pretty much a sheltered existence, and never having been anywhere other than Australia, it was amazing to me to find someone with such interests in common.

I discovered other communities in the fandom, and through my own stories, I began to make a lot of online friends. Writing saved my sanity. My online friends would also tell me I was a talented writer and write encouraging comments.

"Why aren't you doing this professionally?" some would ask.

"Well, actually," would be my usual response before telling them I'd written 300 pages of a novel, which was mostly just scenes I'd come up. I'd started writing the novel in the mid-90s, around the time I was working at the Chronicle, but had never got around to finishing it.

Two very special women refused to let me give up on myself, and encouraged me to finish the novel. One of them rather sternly ordered me to drop everything else, and spend some time finishing the novel. So, I did. Over one summer, I wrote as much as I could in my spare time. It took three months and left a few disappointed 'fans' of my fanfiction, but I completed it. I duly sent it off to my friends to edit and published it a little over a year later.

Those two women I now consider close friends and they continue to keep me going even when I feel like giving up. I have even gone over to the United States to meet them in person. There are others I communicate with regularly, who do not criticise when I vent online, knowing it is a good way to let out my frustrations and gives me strength.

My fanfiction writing has been fairly prolific. I continue to write mostly in the one fandom, although I do have a few stories in other fandoms.

Frustratingly, I have been in and out of employment since

leaving my job as a reporter. I have worked in customer service/call centres and worked as a sub-editor. Most of the time, I feel I have been taken advantage of. The jobs have not been high-paying and in many ways, I have felt I have not been paid my worth.

Call centre work and customer service is probably the worst kind of employment for someone in my position. While I have had some great customers, there have been a minority who have called me 'stupid' or screamed abuse at me because I will not go against company policy.

One particular role was supposedly a temporary position, but I was there for more than two years. My responsibilities far exceeded the brief given to the agency I was contracted to, yet those responsibilities were never recognised in remuneration.

The company I was temping for was part of a bigger operation and had well over 100 employees, many of whom would pass my desk on the way to the kitchen. Some of these people would comment to me about my conversations with customers. It was a fairly open space, and the kitchen was next to my desk, so other employees could hear at least my side of it.

It was often rather worrying to have other people hear these conversations, especially because the sound carried, and we had concrete floors. I admit I did not deal well with customers abusing me and it was evident in the way I would talk to them. I found this increasingly stressful.

When the stress was at its worst, my depression would come back almost full force. I would break down in the middle of the office. I often did not take my morning or afternoon breaks and felt guilty for taking my lunch break because there was often no one to cover for me.

In my last few months there, the stress increased tenfold. We had a new product which proved hugely popular, tripling my workload. My manager hired some more temps to ease the load, but it did not help. What galled was I learnt that the temps, contracted to another agency, were getting paid more than I was. Adding insult to injury, I was not only expected to train them, but supervise them as well. I was angry over this and various other slights through the time I was there and eventually resigned.

Yet, there were times when I handled the stress a lot better and it was noticeable. Everyone I worked with knew I was a writer at heart. They would even comment on it. "You've been writing. You're not nearly as stressed."

Despite the problems in those customer service jobs, I coped well enough to do my job and become very good at it. So much that I had comments like: "Why aren't you managing this place? You know your job better than (so and so)."

Which is rather the point. Despite my depression and despite the stress, I have been able to demonstrate that I can do the job and do it well.

Being under-valued added to the stress and diminished my self-worth. When you are paid less than what you feel the job is worth, it undermines your self-worth.

Less than six months after leaving Auckland to move back to Hamilton, I was hired as a casual sub-editor. For the first time in a very long time, I had found a job that not only I felt more than competent at, but I had co-workers who were so incredibly understanding and the best people I have ever worked with. Sadly, the job was over after a year when the company decided to outsource the work normally given to my team.

I scored a temping role with another company. It was a very small operation, but again, I worked with some very understanding people who knew I had depression but didn't care. I was able to do the job I had been hired for, and that was all they cared about.

I applied for other journalism roles, as it is where I feel the most valued, but have not been able to return to it.

I have been out of paid work since mid-2017. I have lost count of the jobs I have applied for. I have had well-meaning advice from some people who feel that I should be applying for anything out there, whether it is working for a fast-food restaurant or cleaning. I would have difficulty even getting in the door of such jobs because of my skills. I was once told to try for work at a mushroom farm, but the owner took one look at my CV and told me he wouldn't hire me because as soon as something better came along, I would quit. I have been told to omit things from my CV, but I doubt even that would work because of my experience. The fact is, I am competing against far younger people with less experience or education, and it is understandable why employers would not even bother to interview me.

I have had several arguments with my brother over this as well. "Why don't you apply to a supermarket?" he has asked. This is something he has 'suggested' many times, yet he never seems to hear me when I tell him that I have already applied for such roles, only to never be granted an interview. He also seems to think I can just apply for roles that are well below my qualifications, as if it is that easy. I am not the type of person who would be happy working in such a role. For one, I am an intellectual person and that means I need something that is mentally stimulating. Two, I do not want to go backwards in my depression, and to take on any job, just to have enough money coming in, will inevitably cause that backwards slide.

It also feels that he does not see any value in the things I have achieved. In many ways, I think he is a lot like our father, in that in my perspective, he does not value my education. I do not know if that is truly the case or if he is speaking out of concern for the financial stress I am under, but since he does not seem to listen when I try to tell him exactly how I feel, there is little opportunity to talk frankly.

I do wonder if it is not just the fact I am over-qualified for the jobs being advertised, but my mental health history has also had something to do with it - not that I have ever admitted that to a prospective employer. I do have a problem with application forms that ask about health issues. If I say I have no health issues, I would consider it a lie.

I have heard stories of others who have applied for jobs only for the prospective employer to refuse to hire them because of their mental health issues.

There is still a stigma around mental illness that can lead employers to think a person with the illness is incompetent or incapable. That could not be further from the truth.

Chapter Nine: Thoughts of Suicide

There were a few instances where I was close to chucking it all in. I remember, not long after my father passed away, lying in bed one night. I had a bottle of Diazepam in the bathroom cabinet, and I seriously thought about swallowing the pills. Yet a voice stopped me, telling me to hang on.

When I was working for one company, we were doing shift work which involved 40 hours in four days. The shifts were almost impossible to keep up with, spending two days working from 5.30 in the morning to four in the afternoon, then two days working from four in the afternoon to 2.30 in the morning, then four days off. It was gruelling, and I wasn't the only person feeling stressed from such a pattern.

I had a bad depressive episode during my time at this job. It became so bad that a friend took me to the doctor and got her to put me on extended sick leave, then took me to stay at her place for a few days just so I could get my head straight. I remember feeling suicidal then. I was also put on Prozac and it helped take the edge off, but I did not want to take it for too long.

I hated that job.

I have had a few more episodes since then where I have considered it. Thankfully, I have not done more than think of it.

I don't like to think of suicide as a 'selfish' thing to do, although I have heard some people do feel that way. I heard an interview with a celebrity who said he had thought of it, but he felt it was a selfish thing to do because of his family. I get that.

I know of one family who has lost a member to suicide. We can only assume the reasons behind it, and it has been difficult for all, especially because there were young children involved.

There have been times when I have broken down and told my family I felt they were better off without me. Their reactions are mixed, from: "Don't think like that", to "Don't be stupid." I don't think they fully realised just how bad it could get. My mother now understands, but I think my brother still isn't quite there yet.

Here are my thoughts on suicide: for the person going through it, they are trying to end their own pain. From my perspective, it is the feeling or thought that the world would be better off without me. As I may have said, I have often felt that my birth caused problems in my family, and given my father's attitude toward me, I think it was a natural conclusion to come to.

For someone who is suicidal, while I can only offer my perspective, when we are deep within these thoughts, we are unable to see the big picture, or how it would cause others pain.

I am fortunate that I have been able to get that perspective. One of the things that has stopped me is the thought of what it would do to my family and friends. My online friends have been wonderful in their unwavering support.

I am fairly certain that had it not been for the writing and the friends I made, I would not still be here. My friends continue to keep me fighting.

There's a song in a movie I once saw, adapted from a book by Carrie Fisher, who battled many demons for years until her untimely death at the age of 60, and an actress and woman I admired. She was far from perfect but she kept battling on. The movie? **Postcards from the Edge**. The song is sung by Shirley MacLaine, and there is a line in it that illustrates exactly what I say above: *Good times and bad times, I've seen 'em all, but my dear, I am still here.*

For all the crap I have gone through, I am still here. I have had moments where I have battled thoughts of suicide, feelings of utter worthlessness, but my dear, I am still here.

Chapter Ten: Post Hoc Ergo Propter Hoc

Through a lot of self-analysis, and a lot of research, I have been able to work out strategies to cope with my illness. It is far from a perfect system and I consider myself a work-in-progress.

One of the problems I still face is my social anxiety. When I was working, I did not find it easy to make friends. Being unable to take part in social events, either because I chose not to drink, or because of exclusion from such things, made it difficult for me to let my guard down and allow people to get to know me on a more personal level.

There were also times when I hesitated to initiate a casual conversation with my colleagues. Even to the point of not greeting them if we were both in the office kitchen at the same time. I found that difficult, probably because I was taught not to speak unless spoken to. I would often wait until my colleague was finished with whatever they were doing instead of engaging with them. I doubt they ever understood that and perhaps thought I was being anti-social, although I am sure some of them realised I had social anxiety.

To this day, I am still very nervous in social situations and tend not to talk unless it is a subject I know something about and feel I can contribute. It is something I am still working on.

Another problem is my weight. Growing up, I was very skinny. I started putting on weight in my mid-20s, around the time the depression worsened, along with debilitating migraines. At my skinniest as an adult, I was about 50 kilograms.

For my height, 1.64 metres, that was very skinny indeed.

I did not have the best of diets. When I was four, I decided I wasn't going to eat my vegetables, even though I had previously been a fairly good eater. I still have no idea what prompted it, but I have had difficulty ever since. My parents told me that I announced: "I don't want my veggies." My father said: "Well, just eat your meat and potatoes then." That was pretty much my diet from then on.

Did he do the wrong thing? Possibly. There might have been better ways to handle it.

My theory is that I either was told something by another child that led to my behaving that way, or I discovered something that prompted it. My parents did have a vegetable garden, and since I had a phobia when it came to slugs and snails, I may have seen them in the vegetables. The true reason remains a mystery, but I did figure out I had a phobia to the point that if I tried to eat vegetables, I would feel nauseated and would dry-retch.

I ate a lot of junk food as a teenager, yet I compensated for it by exercise - either cycling or walking. At university, I was eating mince pies, potato chips and other fried foods, but the campus was more than nine kilometres from home, so it gave me plenty of exercise.

When I moved to Whangarei, and back in with my parents, I stopped cycling. Part of that was due to my dad, who didn't want me cycling, thinking I couldn't handle the traffic. Dad, of course, was being over-protective, since I had been cycling since I was a kid and didn't have any confidence issues on the bicycle.

The weight began to pile on, and by the time I reached my 40s, I was creeping up toward 90 kilograms. At age 44, I reached 95 kilograms.

I had body issues. I had large breasts, and I hated it. I believe this was a genetic thing, as my grandmother was also big-chested, but my weight certainly didn't help. I am very sensitive about these things and at times can barely say the word breast, let alone anything else. I was once in a bathroom at work checking my reflection in the mirror, pleased I was able to wear a shirt I hadn't been able to wear because of my chest. I had managed to lose a bit of weight, so the shirt was fitting better. A colleague came in and was staring at me as I gazed at my reflection and I told her I hadn't been able to wear the shirt.

"Well, that's because you've got such big tits!"

I hate that word. When people remarked on my size, I would feel so embarrassed and humiliated that I would picture grabbing a knife and just cutting them off. I could never tell people not to talk about them that way.

A breast reduction was my only option, but to get it done privately was a lot of money.

I tried telling my GP in Auckland how it made me feel, but I was often told my chances of getting the surgery were slim. I would have had to pay for the operation myself as it wasn't available then on the public system unless the problem was so bad it was debilitating. I was not considered a priority, even though it was affecting my mental health.

I had heard of some people who managed to get help through charitable organisations. I could not understand why those people got help, but I seemed to always be left in the cold. It was something I questioned frequently. I would ask for help but never got it, putting it down to luck. In fact, I have a saying: "If it weren't for bad luck, I'd have no luck at all".

When I moved to Hamilton, I begged my GP to help me even going so far as to tell him about my thoughts. I believe doing so pushed my case over the line from rejection into potential surgery. I was given an appointment at Waikato Hospital to see the plastic surgeon.

Initially, he declined to do the surgery. He told me I needed to lose weight, a lot of weight, to get my BMI (Body Mass

Index) down to a manageable level. It was too dangerous otherwise. I felt he doubted my ability to lose the weight. I came away from that meeting determined to prove him wrong. I had six months.

I did my best to eat healthily. I still made a lot of mistakes, but having got over many of my past problems with vegetables, I was able to eat some, like lettuce and cherry tomatoes and create a salad of sorts. I learnt to love corn-on-the-cob – not the easiest kind of food for the system but as far as I was concerned it was a vegetable, so it was acceptable. I banned sweets, chocolate and potato chips from my diet.

It was a struggle, especially around Christmas, when I was unable to eat one of my favourite desserts – pavlova. However, I managed to lose 10 kilograms in just over three months. With Easter, I struggled. I freely admit I love chocolate and I did buy Easter eggs. I still managed to keep the weight off.

The thing they don't tell you about dieting is how damn hard it is to do it on your own. You have no one to pull you up and remind you of why you're doing it. You have no one to yell at you to "put that bag of chips down!". You need a lot of self-discipline, and when you've eaten badly for most of your life, it is very, very hard to get that discipline. Yet, always at the forefront of my mind was that goal. That determination to show the surgeon I could lose the weight. I deserved that surgery.

So, even with a few slip-ups, I worked at it. I was working full-time and had the opportunity to take a walk every day during my lunch break. It was enough. By my next appointment, I had lost the required amount of weight. For that, my surgeon congratulated me and told me I deserved the reduction surgery.

The next few months were a waiting game. My weight fluctuated, never going above 84 kilograms, thankfully, and by the time the surgery was booked in mid-November, I had managed to get my weight down to 77 kilograms. The surgery was done and for me, personally, it was the best thing I ever did.

My weight still yo-yos, but I keep working at it.

While my eating is not perfect, I have learnt a few things through the change in diet. My moods have become more stable.

I am not prone to frequent depressive episodes. I still get stressed, especially over money, but it is not pulling me down as much as it used to.

Much of my dietary knowledge has come through research. I subscribed to a number of online systems. If there is one thing I have learnt through study for my first degree, it is to read everything I can get my hands on then form my own opinion. I have taken the information all these dietary 'experts' have presented and used what works for me. I choose not to punish myself for my slips, but make myself work a little harder next time.

I have learnt to be philosophical about food; that it is okay to have something 'unhealthy' from time to time, as long as you don't go overboard.

I also get a bit of exercise when I can. While joining a gym is helpful, it is not always the best thing for some. I prefer going on long walks, or out on the bicycle. It has the added benefit of getting fresh air and a change of scenery instead of looking at a wall while walking on a treadmill or watching something on television. Yes, they are distractions, but not as good.

Sometimes it helps to go walking with someone. They may walk faster than you, which helps you work a little harder and they can not only provide companionship but motivation as well.

I choose not to use medication. I have been on medication in the past and do not find it helpful. I would rather use a course of multi-vitamins. However, this is my preference.

I have a female cat. I have always been a cat person, but it has not always been possible to have a pet, due to my living situation. My cat is very affectionate (when she wants to be, like all cats) and is great for when I need a pick-me-up. Having been without one for a long time, I noticed when I first got her that I became much calmer. I still have my occasional issues, but not as many as when I didn't have her.

I am well aware there will be more episodes in the future and times when I will struggle. I now describe my depression as an old friend; one who is not necessarily welcome, but I will indulge for a little while until I feel it's fine to kick out again.

I was once told not to 'label' myself. I find myself asking why? We label many things. A container of flour we store in the pantry. Clothing. Shoes. Some of us live by labels. Whether they're Manolo Blahniks or Basics. Does it mean one thing is better than the other? In some ways, yes, but it doesn't always mean it's a bad thing. It's simply a way of identifying something.

I once saw something on Facebook. If we could show our illnesses as many with physical symptoms do, we would not be judged as something to be avoided. I have often said if there was a badge for being a battler of depression, I would wear it proudly.

I am not ashamed of it. I refuse to hide what I am. It is as much a part of me as my writing. Is that labelling myself?

To some, knowing I have this illness is reason enough to place me in the 'too hard' basket. They would rather avoid me or skirt around the issue than face it head-on.

To me, by giving myself this 'label', it shows that I am a survivor.

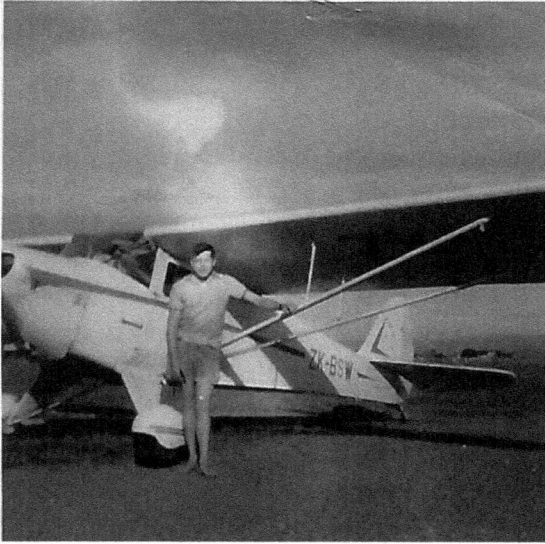

Dad, some time in the 1960s. He had a private pilot's licence although he stopped flying long before I was born.

Mum, in her teens. I'm told I look a lot like her.

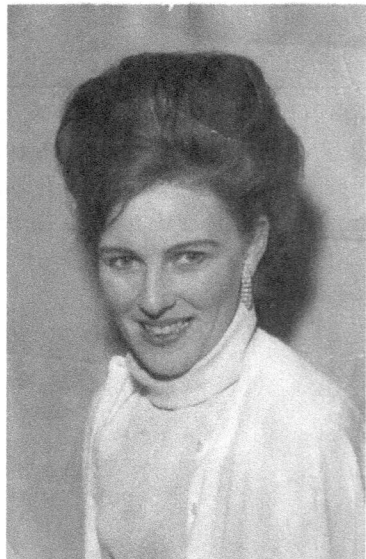

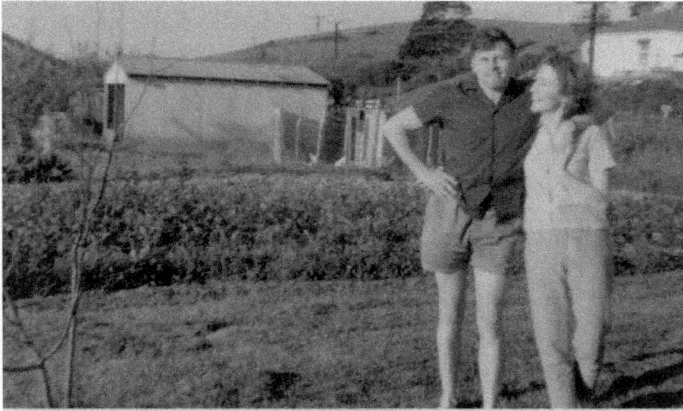

Mum and Dad, before my brother and I came along.

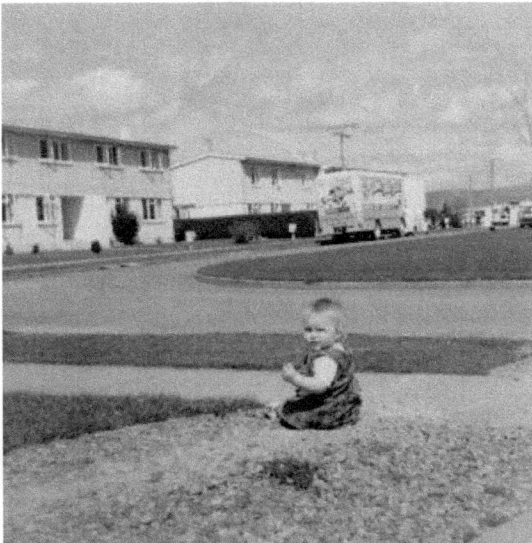

I was about two, caught eating stones on the driveway in Croydon Ave.

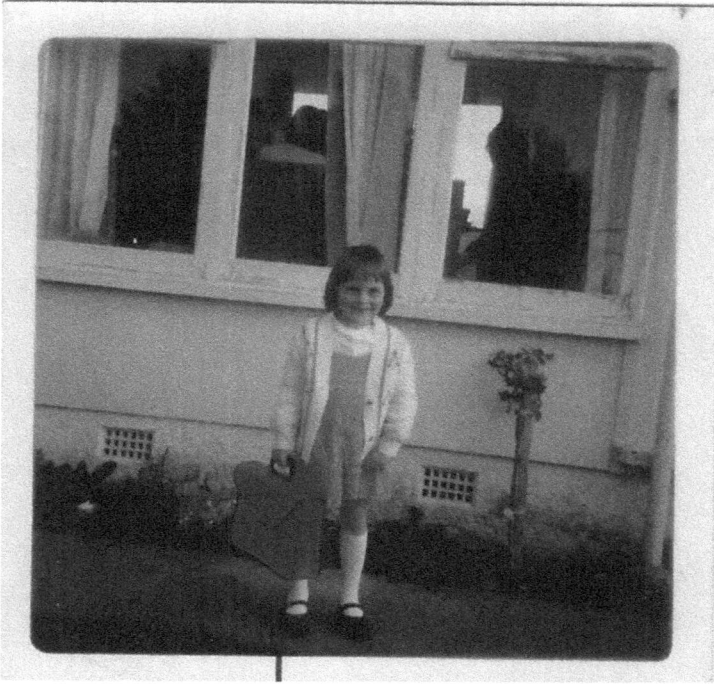

My fifth birthday. I was so excited to be
going to school with my brand new (orange)
bag.

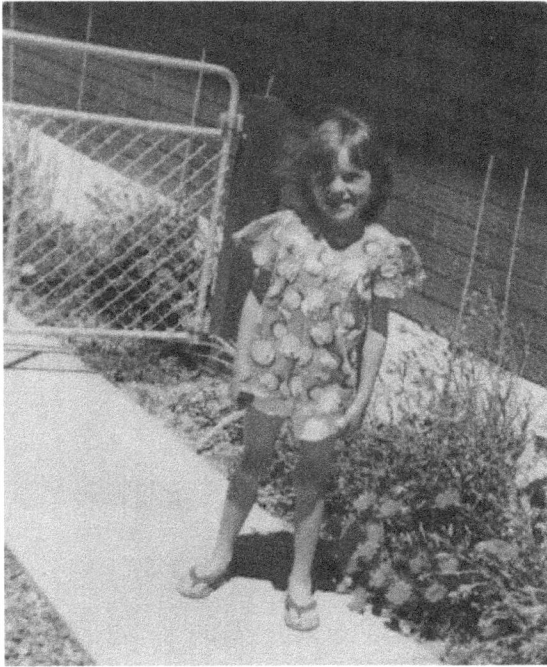

I must be about 6 or 7 as it was before I started wearing glasses and enough time had passed for the plants to grow. There was nothing along the side of the house when we moved in October 1976.

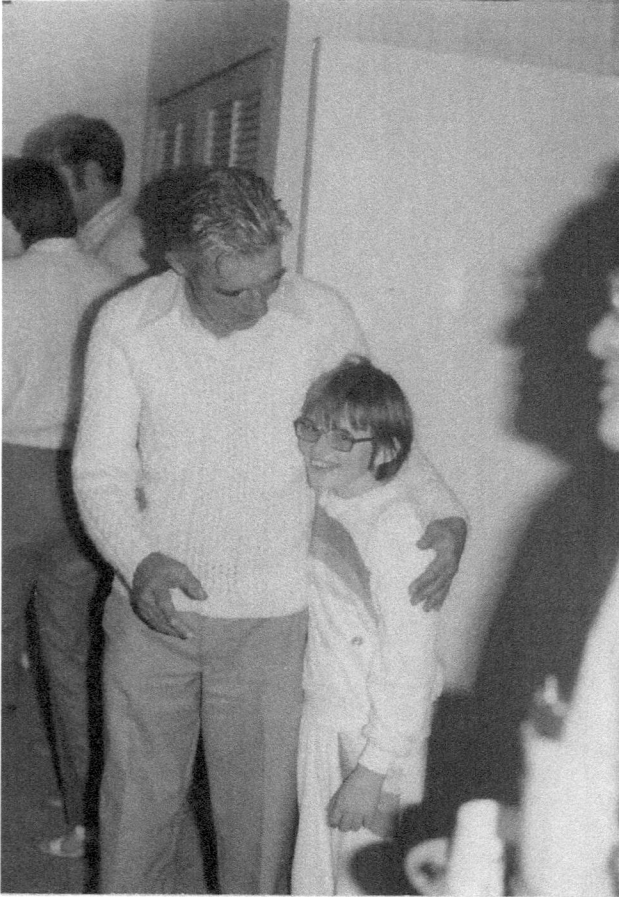

Me with Grandad Carroll when I was about 10. I adored
him and according to my Mum, it was mutual. He was a
good-natured man with a great sense of humour.

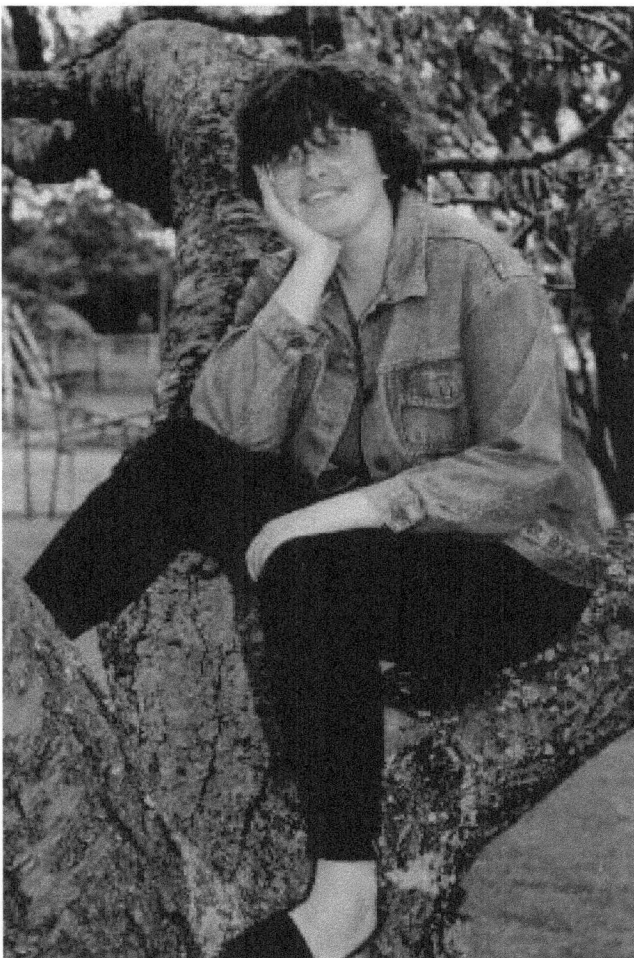

One of the photographers at the Levin Chronicle was trying to use up some colour film so she took a few pics of me. Photo: Jan Rolston

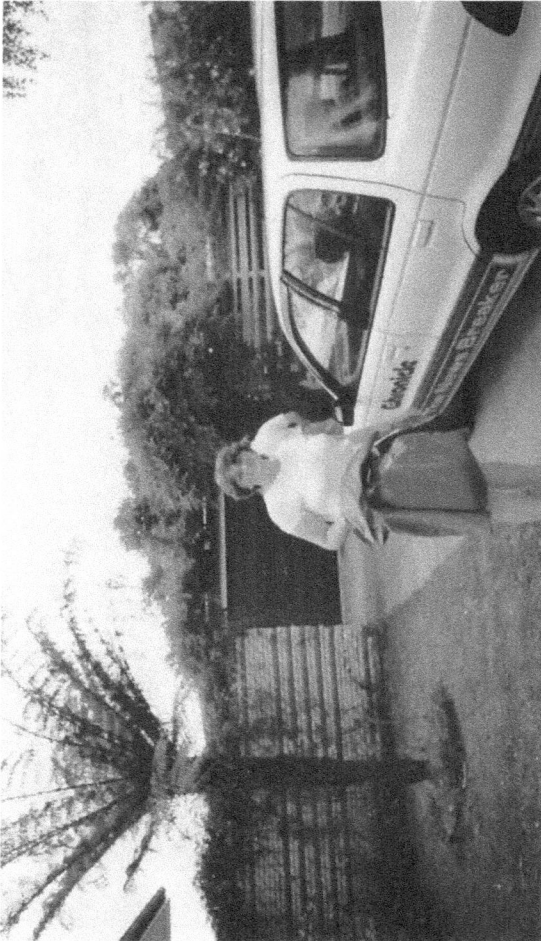

1997 – This is when my chest started getting noticeably bigger.

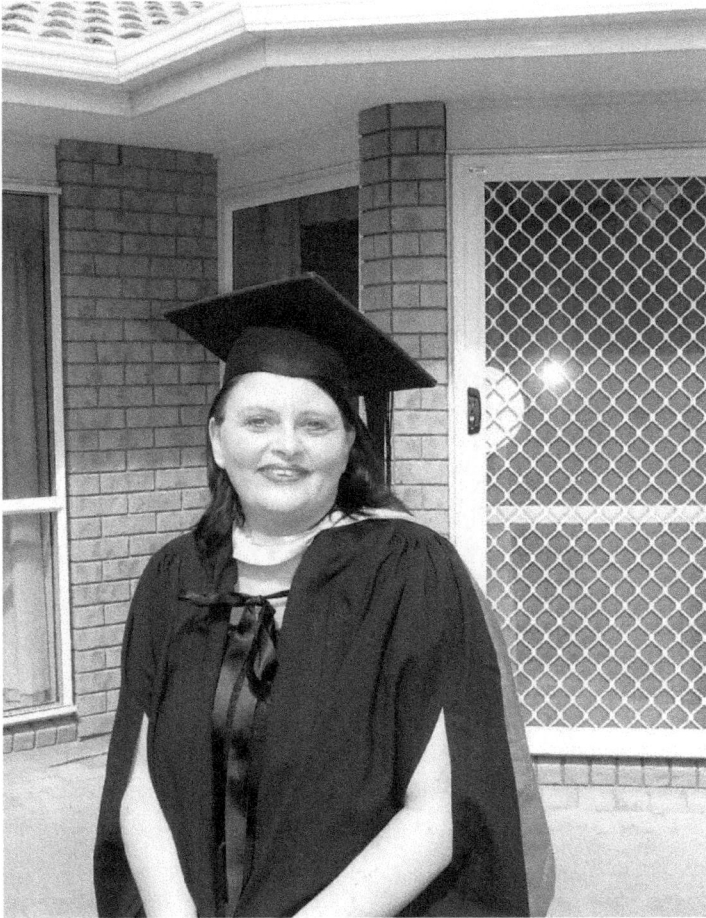

I had wanted to get a professional photo done for my graduation from AUT in 2007 but couldn't afford it, so this was taken at my Mum's home in Hamilton. I didn't go to my graduation the first time, so this was a big deal for me.

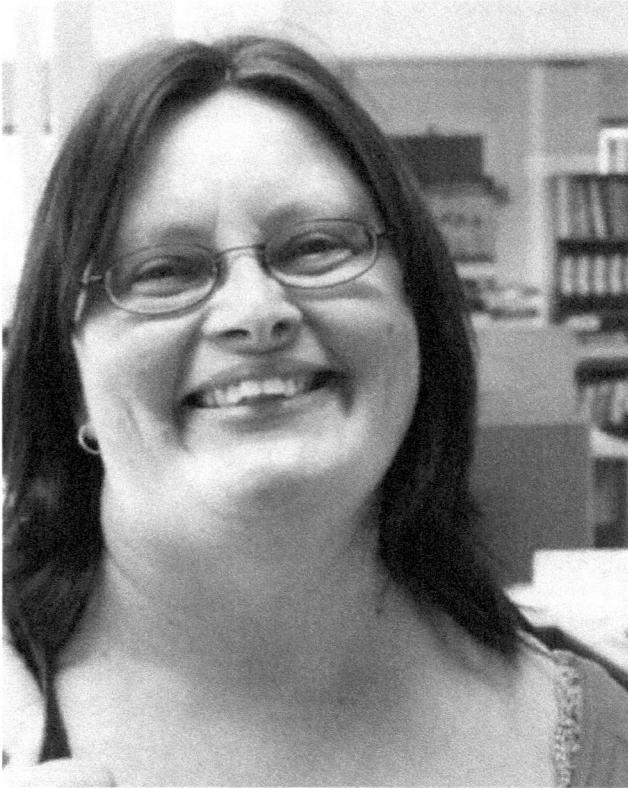

Taken at the Western Leader by a colleague. My
teeth look worse in this photo.

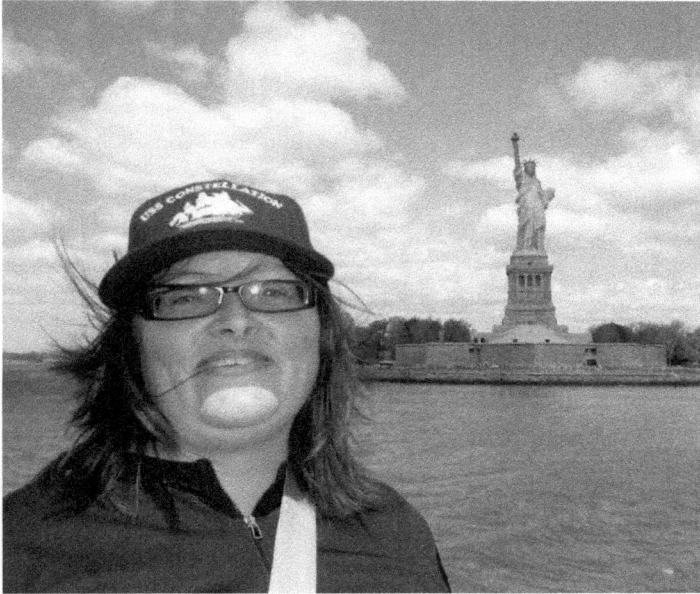

May 2013, on the Hudson River in New York. It was
the first holiday I'd ever taken by myself, further
afield than Australia.

Section Two: Stories

These are stories others have shared with me about their own experiences and things they may have learnt which help them through their depression. Some names have been changed.

Chapter Eleven: Ray

Waking up in a hospital bed, in a full brace, wondering what had happened was the one thing that led me to where I am today. Lying in that bed, with only my thoughts to keep me company, worrying if I was ever going to walk again, was probably one of the lowest points of my life.

I'd been at rock-bottom before, but I'd managed to get through.

That day had been the culmination of about a year of problems. But those problems began much earlier.

It started when I was young, before I was eight. My parents split when I was about four or five, but then my mother met a guy and got remarried. That marriage eventually fell apart, and that was probably the beginning for me. I didn't know then it was depression, and I wasn't diagnosed until I was an adult.

Mum was what I would call a functional alcoholic. It may have been genetic. My grandma was a heavy drinker. As a kid, I didn't think she had a drinking problem, but she always had a glass of whiskey, and she was seated a lot. My grandfather also began drinking heavily, but I never saw him as an alcoholic. My uncle once asked him: "Why do you drink all the time?" Grandma had passed away by this time, and he said: "If I had not, she would have drunk it all." He rarely drank when she was gone, so he did it for her. He felt he had to help because if he hadn't, she would have just kept going and going.

My stepfather was an alcoholic in the sense that he was the sort of guy who would get himself to a certain level and stay there all day. The whiskey would be sitting on the fridge, and he would go and do what he did, then go to the fridge, take a couple of sips, put it back and just continue. He'd never get severely drunk.

I had quite a messy childhood because of Mum's alcoholism. She was always making mistakes. She said before she passed away that she had always been really selfish in life. The sad thing is, I never got to find out why she did the things she did. I do think she was severely depressed and medicated with alcohol.

Mum was an awesome lady, and we did have some good times, some funny moments, some dramas, but she was really not a good example.

We lived in Wainuiomata and life was good, but then Mum's marriage broke up, and we moved to the Hutt Valley, and that's where it started to turn bad.

We lived in the poorest areas where the rents were cheaper. I tended to gravitate toward the naughty kids, doing naughty things. Mum didn't really know what we were up to as she wasn't paying attention.

I started stealing: burglarising stores, getting involved in armed hold-ups. It got very bad, and it felt like I was being something I wasn't. I didn't really have the heart to do that sort of thing. It probably made my depression worse because I was doing things that only made me feel guilty. I was bringing home stuff that I'd stolen and even began stealing to order. Stealing cars and that sort of thing.

It was when I got arrested for drunk driving that I hit rock-bottom. I'd been arrested before, but this time seemed to be different.

I was four times the legal limit. I'd drunk two forty-ounce bottles of Jim Beam straight and a dozen beers, then got in the car to drive to my mate's place and got pulled over. From that moment, sitting in the back of the police car, going to the station, being processed, knowing the policemen there, them knowing me, I just felt tired. That was more or less the start of the change.

The first time I'd been caught drunk driving, I was sent to jail for three months. I tried really hard not to drink when I got out, but I started drinking again, and got caught again. I was given an option: go back to jail or go to Rehab. I chose Rehab and went to stay at a rehabilitation centre.

When I was there, I made every effort. I was supposed to be in there for eight weeks, but after six weeks they asked me if I wanted to stay for ten. I agreed, but then I got into an argument with another resident and packed my bags and left. I'd already done my time as far as the staff were concerned, but they were worried, so when they found me they told me I was more than welcome to go back anytime I needed them.

For ten years, I didn't touch any alcohol. I began straightening out, working and paying off a mountain of debt I'd accrued.

I'd had a son by this time, and I focused on him, making a point of being in my son's life, despite some difficulties with his mother.

Then, one day when I was 28, a work colleague took me aside. He must have noticed a few things, so he called me into the office.

"I don't mean to pry," he said. "I suffer from depression and I think you do, too."

He told me to go online and take this test, answering questions, then to take the form to my doctor. The doctor looked at the results.

"This is all the questions I would have asked you," he told me. "These are the answers I need."

He then told me he thought I had depression. I just thought I was having a bad run, or that it was just life. It was a relief that it had a name and that it was something real. It wasn't me or my imagination. I no longer felt damaged.

I'd often asked myself: "What have I done in a previous life to put me in this position to feel this bad every day for all these years."

After a few years I ended up in Otaki, met my daughter's mother and started over. Then that relationship fell apart, and I ended up drinking again. I drank heavily for about a year until I was in a car accident with some friends. The crash killed the driver, and I ended up in hospital.

Following my discharge from hospital, I started slipping back into depression again. I'd go and rent a ton of movies and just lie on the couch and watch movie after movie for three months. My rent got behind, and I had to move. I'd needed to have an operation to fix my arm, which had been snapped in the accident, and I was missing hospital appointments.

I'd stayed with friends and family, but even that didn't help when we'd end up having arguments. By the time I did have the operation I was living in a caravan at my dad's, on painkillers, staying up all night listening to talkback radio and sleeping all day. I was bored, writing stuff in a journal that was just too depressing. It was meant to be a journal for my daughter, but everything I was writing was horrible.

Things began to slowly improve. I did seek counselling but realised it wasn't for me.

There have been times that I have had suicidal thoughts. Someone once told me suicide is quitting; it's giving up, and I don't want to do that. My son's birth was a big catalyst for me. I had those thoughts, but I didn't want to leave him and for him having to tell people: "Where's your dad?" "Oh, he killed himself." The thought of that depressed me even more, so I just held on.

I used to resent the way my mother raised me. As I got older, I realised parents can only work with the tools they have and if they're not willing to get new tools and happen to be stuck in their way, it's what they have.

After my mother passed away from throat cancer, I moved and took a job as a storeman. I'd been a chef before, over the last fifteen years. Even through the crimes I was committing, I was still working. I stopped working as a chef because I didn't have any spare time. Working in my current job suits me, and I'm happy now. I work for six hours and restore furniture at home for extra money.

I've never hidden my depression. I think people need to know because it's pretty common. The thing about depression is, you can't see it. For people to understand, it has to be something tangible. It has to be there, able to be seen or touched.

It's hard though because no one really takes notice of us, but once a famous person stands up, it becomes less taboo - it's like that #MeToo campaign. That's been going on for how long? How many hundreds of years? And then, because a couple of celebrities stand up and say yeah, it's become something, it's not cool.

After my last really bad bout of depression, I slipped badly. I didn't want to go back on medication, so after sitting in that depressed state for about six months, which is too long, I decided that I was not going to let it get me. The friends I stayed with after the accident helped me get off the medication, and it was just through being active - active in their Marae, or their family, that I got better.

When those thoughts start creeping in, they will come in and sit there, and it will click in my mind: "I know what this is, this is the depression trying to latch on again." So then I'd take steps to combat it.

One of the handiest things for me was working on the car or

on the motorbike - doing something that I could use to focus my mind; something I know how to do that I'm good at. While I'm working on it, sometimes I'd play YouTube clips; uplifting clips of people who have done good things with their lives and been through depression. Sometimes it's not about someone with depression but just people who have gone through hard times in their lives.

There was one guy in particular who had a severe learning disability, so his brain wasn't 100 per cent functional. The main story was that he is now extremely functional in his mind - he's known for it and he teaches people how to memorise things and how to use their brain. He was made fun of at school because he wasn't the quickest or the brightest.

Hearing these people, I used to think: 'Man, I've got it tough', but then I listen to these stories and realise they've had it tougher and managed to get through it. It's not about getting out there and being known all over the world. You can be chatting to someone at work and lifting them up a bit, or people you know who aren't feeling the best, and you're lifting them up.

I feel good making people feel good, and that's how I get around it.

It's always going to be there; it's just catching it when it hits me and not letting it consume me.

At the peak of it, it is hard to change the thinking, because you're in it. I just ride it out until I get to a point where I can deal with it. Once I notice it, start locking myself away or playing video games for days on end or something like that, I know I'm stuck, and then I need to do something.

Sometimes my methods might change. I might discover new things or a new passion or something. Sometimes it takes someone to say to me: "You all right, bro?" And I'm like: "Yeah. Oh, actually, no, I'm not." They can see from the outside I'm not my usual self. That's another way I can catch it as well.

Nowadays I don't let it sit around too long. I can usually catch it and push it out. There's always a way, but sometimes you get trapped in that 'woe is me' thing. I learned something in rehab: 'Poor me, poor me, pour me another'. That's something that's always stuck in my mind. When I start getting the poor mes, I think: 'Well no, not poor me'. I'm strong enough to deal with whatever this is. Let's do it. But catching it's the thing.

I tend to think, I've done it before, I can do it again. I have to remember that.

Chapter Twelve: Judith

Twenty-two. It's not even my favourite number. If I hadn't dropped pill number 23, who knows how many I would have taken. Who knows if I would be here to share my story?

When that antidepressant clattered on the floor, I rang 111. All I had wanted was to stop the physical and mental pain I was in. My brain was telling me there was no other way. No hope. My neck felt like it had a tonne of concrete injected into it. I didn't want to leave my bed. I slept a lot, but each time I turned over was hard work. Going to the toilet was my Everest. Even though I have the most amazing friends, I honestly thought no one cared. Even the need to care for my cat – which had pulled me through on many an occasion – didn't kick in.

I'd tried the Mental Health Crisis Team and told them I couldn't get out of bed. They said it was a physical problem and to ring my GP. I'd tried my self-described partner, but he said he was at work. I managed to make an appointment with my GP but I couldn't hold on. I needed to stop the mental anguish and physical aching then and there.

So that's how I ended up in the A and E waiting room one winter Thursday afternoon. Even though I'd arrived by ambulance, there was no room for me in A and E proper. So I sat – me, whose face had appeared in tens of thousands of mailboxes for nearly six years, some might say a public figure – in a nightgown and coat, no underwear. I hadn't had a shower since the Sunday and could barely see through my glasses, they were so tear stained.

I didn't care. It's only now, when I think back, what a wreck I must have looked. I just remember feeling incredibly spacey.

When the crisis team finally got to me at 1.45am, they said I would be referred to a psychiatrist. Instead, someone else rang me the next day and said I was discharged into the care of my GP. My GP was shocked.

My father used to call me Hour in the Shower, after a racehorse no less. Yet, showering and brushing my teeth were the first things to go when my depression got worse. I've often thought people with depression and/or anxiety should get a subsidy for their subsequent fillings.

I was diagnosed with depression when I was 29. I was doing what I'd wanted to since I was about 11, studying journalism. I can't recall the symptoms that prompted me to go to the doctor, but I later found out two of my tutors were also battling depression.

I suspect my depression first manifested when I was a teenager. I would spend a lot of time on my bed crying, staring at the flowers-in-baskets-patterned wallpaper I'd chosen. While my brother and I had been close, things changed when I was sent to boarding school. When it was his turn to go to boarding school, he refused. He appeared to resent my visits home every three weeks that disrupted his only child set-up. At his wedding, he apologised for the way he had treated me, and my mother later described it as him 'knocking the stuffing' out of me. For my final two years of secondary school, I returned home and went from a 120-student, single-sex school to a 1000-plus co-ed school. I was bullied by some younger students as they thought I was the sister of another student they were already bullying.

I had about four attempts to wean myself off the depression medicine. Two were utter failures. I made a passive attempt at suicide while driving the work car home one night. It was a windy road, and I'd keep closing my eyes hoping I'd drift into another car, a tree – anything to end the pain. Something made me open my eyes and then I would close them again.

The second, utter failure, was my first panic attack. I didn't know what was happening. I rang a taxi to take me to the doctors, but my breathing was so bad the lovely taxi phone operator rang an ambulance and stayed on the line until it arrived. I couldn't stop crying. I was escorted into the side door to wait for the next available doctor. It was my GP who had encouraged me to go off my medication even though I wasn't convinced.

My last panic attack was on the floor outside the toilets of my favourite café. I was lucky that the woman who came to my aid knew what to do to get my breathing under control again.

I was named after a relative of my mother's, who had hung herself in a tree in the backyard of the family home when she was 19. I was born on the 19th. Her mother had made numerous suicide attempts and spent time in a psychiatric hospital.

My paternal grandfather killed himself; one of his daughters attempted suicide.

Yet, there was no discussion about looking after one's mental health in our family.

When I turned 19, I thought to myself: "What now, do I kill myself?" About the only time my father ever told me off was when I was in my late 20s, and I said to my mother I thought it was a stupid idea to name a child after someone who had killed themselves.

I'd always considered myself lucky – the medication I was prescribed worked, and I had no noticeable side effects. After my suicide attempt, I was given a new diagnosis – anxiety – and new medication.

The hardest thing I've found about my periods of mental unwellness has been the two people who are meant to love and cherish me the most – my mother and my partner – made no attempt to understand depression and anxiety and how to help me. My mother is very much of the school of "get out of bed, go do something". If only it was that simple.

However, I have the most amazing friends. Many of them have had their own battles with mental unwellness or seen someone close to them go through it.

I continue to take my anti-anxiety medication and am not aware of any side effects. More importantly, I haven't had a panic attack since.

Exercise is a huge part of how I keep well. I exercise as much for the mental benefits as the physical and weight management benefits.

Having friends who understand anxiety and check in with me regularly is also a major part of my wellness regime.

My advice

If a friend or loved one is living with depression and/or anxiety:

• do some research – Google, read a book, visit a support organisation

• ask your friend or loved one when they are well what help they might need when they are unwell and what help they need to stay well

• check in with them regularly – it can be as simple as an "are you ok" text or reminding them of something they have achieved or what you admire in them

• understand that their getting well could be a long haul

• understand what triggers their anxiety and never push them into those situations. You wouldn't say to a coeliac "go on; you can do it, Nana Pat made this bread just for you" or to someone allergic to peanuts "oh, you are such a drama queen, a few won't hurt you". A happy mind is more important than appearances and a desire to play happy families.

• don't be ashamed of them

• don't underestimate the strength they are using to constantly battle their brain

- don't say "we all have down days"
- offer practical support – cook them a meal, clean their house, do their shopping, wash their dishes, hang out their washing
- just like it is wise to know what to do if someone has a heart attack or starts choking, learn what to do if someone is having a panic attack

Most of all, remember people with depression and anxiety do come out the other side and are often the most loving, caring, creative, intelligent and funny people you will ever meet.

Chapter Thirteen: Claire

I was driving home one day, after dropping the kids at school, having thoughts of doing 'something'. I didn't have a plan, but I had vague ideas of a razor blade and a bath. It was as I began mentally composing a letter to my friends and family, still behind the wheel of my car, that I realised what I was about to do.

I wasn't worried about my children. I knew someone would notice they were still at school and sort them out. I just thought everyone would be better off without me.

I had another friend who had suicidal thoughts, and it was as I was mentally composing the letter to him that it clicked. We'd always promised to tell the other if we ever felt suicidal.

I pulled over, rang my doctor, and I was seen that day.

I was 35 when I was diagnosed with depression. My youngest child had been born, and I didn't bounce back from the depression, that was at its worst during pregnancy, like I had with my other two children.

I went to my doctor and did a test on a pad of paper. I think I was ticking boxes. It was then that I realised it was depression.

I'd known for a long time prior to that test, but I was in denial and refused any offers of help. My midwife, during my third pregnancy, offered to take me for some help, but I told her I was fine.

So, yes, I was in denial for a long time. I felt such a failure and tomorrow would be a better day.

Looking back, I recall specific episodes as a child where I believe depression and anxiety were always underlying, but it hit big time when I reached puberty.

I had no idea what depression was at that age, let alone anxiety. I just thought I was being pathetic and silly.

I dealt with it over the years, but I didn't realise how bad it was until after I was medicated and feeling like the sunshine was back in my life again. Over the years, I'd known others with depression, and I was always amazed that they could get help, but I certainly never clicked that what I had was depression. I just thought I was a grumpy person who had nasty thoughts in my head constantly.

I believe I have had situational depression through my childhood and marriage, but there is also an underlying or maybe overriding imbalance there somewhere.

I have had other low points in my depression. While I felt good I had asked for help after that first incident, and had been able to get that help, I had told my now ex-husband, who only had critical comments instead of supportive ones. Having the benefit of hindsight, I now realise I was in an abusive marriage. However, I continued to stay in that relationship for another nine years.

I chose to end my marriage not long after I had another period of suicidal thoughts. I knew if I left the house, I would drive in front of a truck, so I dealt with it by not leaving. What had been the catalyst for this was the discovery that my then-husband had been lying to me.

When I informed him of my suicidal thoughts, he was horrified, only to tell me a day or two later that I had merely been attention-seeking as I hadn't attempted anything.

It had gotten to the point where I was sleeping my life away. I would do what had to be done: sort the kids, clean the house to a basic standard and then have a nap, get up, do something and have another nap. I was also looking online, trying to prove I wasn't in an abusive relationship.

I still feel I am a 'work-in-progress'. I believe I always will be. I am still on medication, and this has changed over the years in both what I take and the dosage. I have been through counselling which has helped immensely, and my own journey of becoming a counsellor has helped me with strategies to manage my depression.

I feel as though I was always depressed and anxious, even as a young child. How much is nature and how much is nurture I don't know, but in my case, I believe my personality contributed, but so did my upbringing.

Some of the strategies I use include writing in a journal and taking medication, as well as making sure I get enough sleep. I try to be aware of who is in my life - this is more so since I left my husband and realised how much control I have over who I spend my time with. Time alone is vital self-care.

I've learnt from my depression that I am not just a grumpy, nasty person with nasty thoughts. That I have so much good in me to give, but I need to be well to do this. Self-care is part of that wellness.

My depression does not define me any more than, for example, having arthritis would. It is better to be open and honest that I have depression and anxiety. Not as an excuse but to help explain why I might struggle to go out at times, or why I don't always socialise.

The more open and honest I am about it, the easier I find it to manage my life. People then understand that I'm not being a snob for not turning up on a night out but that I was trying really hard and just couldn't quite get there that night. The nights I did get there, I felt support rather than negative comments by people. For example, a snide: "Oh, you made it this time." I'd get more support such as: "Shall I meet you outside?" or "Would you like me to pick you up?" As others understood, I also understood myself more and what I needed to get by.

Another thing I have learnt is how strong I am. I am still here and no longer think of suicide. I might have fleeting thoughts, but those are just fleeting and never take hold like they once did.

Ironically, I used to be scared to die because I didn't want to die feeling so miserable. While I certainly don't want to die, that fear of dying and feeling miserable has gone.

My ex-husband doesn't believe in depression or anxiety and is not supportive. It took time for me to learn to trust who I could talk to and who I couldn't. It took nine years to inform my dad I have depression and I think if Mum was still alive, I wouldn't have told either of my parents.

I have friends who know, and they're great. Social media is helpful for messaging friends when I need to talk but don't want to use the phone. My new partner doesn't understand depression but tries to understand me and never minimises or dismisses.

Chapter Fourteen: David

I was sitting in my car, having just been confronted by someone while out on a job. The man had gotten in my face, being very abusive. I knew I had to get away from the situation as quickly as possible and got in the car.

I rang my boss and related what had happened.

It was not the first time I'd found myself in a bad situation at work.

It had been bad for a while. Many of my colleagues had left over a period of several months, having lost their jobs due to redundancy. It had almost been a waiting game to see who would be next. People I'd known for years were leaving, but somehow I was promoted. It didn't help my personal situation.

I'd had periods of anxiety from the age of 15, but I didn't see it as leading to depression. Looking back, with a lot of self-analysis, I realise that my depression started in my 20s. I was officially diagnosed about four years ago.

My work was stressful. It wasn't just the redundancies, although watching my colleagues leaving was almost like I was losing my safety net. In many ways, it was like being in an abusive relationship - knowing I was in a bad situation but powerless to leave.

It wasn't really one incident that stands out that led me to feeling I had depression. It began with a general sense of unwellness. Then things came to a head when I realised there were things about my job I would rather avoid doing.

I knew something was wrong. So, I sought help through the depression.org.nz website. While I didn't follow all the suggestions on the site, I did take the test to see if my suspicions were correct. I even took it a few more times, just to be sure.

It was a little like the definition of insanity - doing the same thing over and over and getting the same result.

I went to my GP, but the doctor wasn't helpful, only prescribing an anti-depressant.

I reached out to my general manager. Luckily, I had a manager who was not only understanding but very supportive, giving me time off. As scary as it was telling my manager, I don't know what I would have done if they had been a 'dickhead'.

During that time off, I realised I couldn't do my job anymore, and decided to resign. I took on another role in a similar field, but the stress in that role was just as bad as the other job. I sought advice from my boss, who, as it happened, had also been through depression.

I've tried suicide twice. The first time, or so I was told, I entered a fugue state. All I remember was that I had a knife in my hand and was using it to cut myself.

For my second attempt, I took sleeping pills. These were what I like to call 'horse pills'. It was the stupidest way I could have done it as all it did was make me very sleepy.

It was a major turning point in my life. I had to ask myself if I was going to continue to be dumb or if I was going to fight it.

I found a sense of victory by choosing to follow my own path to wellness, instead of getting help from a health system which really didn't help much at all.

I did some research and picked up a few things about exercise, but I'm a lazy bastard. Structured exercise isn't for me.

I knew I needed regularity and found a job through a friend - something unrelated to what I was doing before. The job means I'm forced to exercise as it involves heavy lifting, but there is also no stress. I've built myself a world where I can combat the depression. I know if I go back to what I was doing before, I will slide backwards.

It has taken time for my family to come to terms with my depression. My mother-in-law is of the generation that didn't talk about depression and feels it is an imaginary illness. My wife grew up being told there is no such thing. It's hard for her to understand it.

I'm luckier than most, in that I have great, supportive friends. Others may mock me but at least I have friends who I want to be around. They might ask weird questions, but the way I deal with that is to talk about it.

I have a mate who is well aware of what I'm going through, and that helps, but sometimes he can be a little over the top (with his concern).

Having depression is a constant battle, but I've got the weapons. I do choose to take medication, and it has taken trial and error to know which is right for me. Others might decide they don't want to use medication, but it's my personal choice, and I'm comfortable with that. I have no desire to come off the pills.

I also spend time doing something I love, like being with my children or taking time out with my friends. The important thing is connecting with someone.

Chapter Fifteen: Kathy

I don't think I was ever actually diagnosed with depression. I probably had post-natal depression when my youngest child was born, but it was never actually diagnosed. I think that was part of the problem. It's like when you know something is wrong, but you don't know how to ask for help and when you do so, you're struggling.

People often don't realise that there's actually something wrong, and they just think you're having a bad day and say: 'You'll be right'.

For me, (depression) is just total exhaustion where it's difficult to get up and do anything. Just making a phone call, getting up and getting dressed in the morning. I put up with that for years. I also had sort of peri-menopause, which was never diagnosed. I had a solid two years of just, total, physical exhaustion, just trying to struggle through and survive day by day.

It's not a sadness, it's just a lack of total emotion. It's like you're living in a fog the whole time. People who know me when I was at my worst said they'd never seen me smile. Now, I can laugh at something and I think that really helps.

People who don't know what depression is like don't understand what you need.

I find I can be very sensitive to noise. If I have the music on, it's usually at a very low-level because that's what I can tolerate.

If I'm in a bad way, I don't need music at all.

When the doctors go through the questionnaire, (trying to determine) how far down you are, they ask something I can never understand: "Do you feel fidgety." When I'm down, I don't want to move. (However), I see that one side of depression is that they can be over-active – they've got a jittery feeling and have to keep moving. I'm the opposite. I just literally have not got the energy, even to stand up and do the dishes.

There is a stigma about mental health. I was brought up with that. My natural mother had a lot of mental health problems. She was very smart, but she had a lot of those problems, or so my stepmother would tell me. If I had a problem, she would say I would end up in Porirua (where there was a psychiatric hospital).

My mother left when I was about six, and my little brother was three. My father was struggling to raise all six of us (I had one older brother and three sisters). He was a quiet sort of man and just wasn't strong enough to deal with it.

My father remarried when I was about nine, and my stepmother took over. She had a very strong personality, but I believe she was also deeply insecure. Our former life was just cut off. We (my brother, who was three years younger, and I) weren't allowed to remember my older brothers and sisters. They were all excluded. She was just so strong, and because I was quiet, like my dad, we just had to cave-in. It became so much a habit that I just shut down and tried to stay out of trouble.

There were times when I would just shut down. I lived in a fantasy world where I could read, because books don't hurt you. There were a lot of times where I felt it would be nice to wake up in a fairy-tale world where I could just wake up in the morning and the whole world would be brand new. The 'Prandsome Hince' (The story of Rindercella, as told on tv show Hee Haw) would be there, and everything would be fine.

I got married very young, at 19. Even when I was engaged, there were times when I was allowed to see my fiancé and times when I wasn't. He would call around during the week, and I would go to my bedroom and not speak to him. That was how strong my stepmother's control was.

Years later, I was still living very close to her, and she would still try to control me, even to the point of not allowing me to have friends. I had an older lady come over to help me get started on my day, and sometimes I would take her to my stepmother's house only for Mum to refuse to speak to her, only asking her questions through me.

She just wanted me in this tight little box. Even when I was married, she was still controlling me. I missed out on a lot. I didn't have the teenage rebellion, and I never learnt to stick up for myself. When I did try to stick up for myself, I didn't know how to do it in a good way.

She never praised me, for anything and was very critical, yet, after I learnt to drive, if she wanted to go somewhere, it was okay for her to use me as a driver.

She was a very strait-laced type of woman who believed people should 'keep their clothes on'. I remember there was one night when we went to the movies and there was a scene in it where the characters were sitting in a truck, and the girl was taking off her top. My stepmother walked out, and we followed her. She refused to be driven home, so she walked.

She could give you the silent treatment. We'd have Christmas Day, and Dad would say to us afterwards: "You know that Mum never spoke to me all day." Dad would be at home on his own, and she would say that he was out, as well. We were never allowed any contact with our own dad on our own.

There's a lot of baggage.

I think I learnt, from a very early age just to withdraw, and shut down. Even my doctor said that it had become so ingrained it would take a lot to change.

It's the paradox of depression. You need a strong support system. But, because I'm so quiet, it's easier for dominant people to take over and I feel smothered. So, I'm still not doing what's right for me. I don't put myself first. I will look after everybody else first - that's what we were taught. Women are there to do the caretaking.

I had a bout of depression around the time my marriage was breaking up – so, of course, the depression was tied with the break-up. I went on very strong anti-depressant medication, but I had the flu and came off it cold turkey.

Then I had panic attacks. It was total fear. I'd be standing in the supermarket getting my groceries, and I would just have to run out of there. I just couldn't stand to be around anybody. I still have it now, being in a strange place. I just feel sick to my stomach and really shaky. I used to get it in the library – a feeling like the ceiling was closing in on me.

My mistake was that I didn't try for help. I just shut down and put up with it. So, it's become normal, like being left-handed or right-handed. That was just my normal day-to-day feeling. I didn't really realise that I did have a problem.

I think I was in survival mode – just existing. It's the only regret I have now, that I've wasted a lot of time.

The trouble is, when you do reach out for help, and you don't get the right kind of help, that makes you withdraw even more. At one stage I had a counsellor that was really good, but for some reason she had to cancel an appointment, and she never followed through to help me restart. It may just have been her problems, but I took it very personally.

I sort of feel like I don't have any self-worth, so I think I'm not important enough to be helped.

I've got my guidelines now. I've learnt to accept sleeping tablets - I always sort of felt that taking medication was a sign of weakness. You should be able to deal with it yourself. I think it is that fear that if I start taking medication then I'm that little bit closer to being put in an asylum. It's that fear of not being let out again. I think I've got that same fear of getting older and getting closer to not being able to look after myself, that is a real scary thought of being put into an old folks' home. There, you don't have that control. I'm a messy brat. There's nobody at home now to control that messiness, there's only me.

I've struggled on my own because I'm scared that if I ask for help I'm going to be made to do something I don't want to do but I'm gonna be too scared to say no, this doesn't work for me. I've read a lot of books.

I've had a couple of really bad jobs where I've lasted in both of them eight years. To have survived through that and still keep going, I've done well for myself. So now, if I want to get fat, sit on my butt and read all day, I'm old enough now to do it.

It's probably only in the last couple of years that I've finally got the job that suits me and by working part-time I can balance it. I actually find I can be in a really bad state on my way to work, but just going to work, just shutting your mind off and doing something normal, doing something that you can actually achieve, that makes things better.

I think that's my support system.

It's only recently I've had that. I've had 30-plus years of depression and now I'm just starting to say: "Okay, this is who I am, I'm okay as I am."

I know I've got my limitations. Sometimes I feel like I'm on the outside of the circle. I've never really had any close friends and part of me would like to be included with everybody else's fun, but then too much of it isn't right for me either.

It's easier to do without than try and struggle with something that's not really good for you.

I've never been suicidal, probably because I don't like pain.

My son once came home with his wife to help look after me, but I see now that it wasn't good for me. It wasn't me being looked after. They were only young, and they didn't understand.

I couldn't support someone else with depression. Someone I know tried to commit suicide, but they got her back. During the period she was really down, I found it difficult to deal with her. It's very hard to be a support person. You can see it on the ads on tv (like those for Depression.org.nz), where they say: "We're here for you." It's very hard for us to explain what we actually need. It's only when we've come out of a bad patch we can see what was good for us and what wasn't.

I don't have very many totally normal days. My depression is extremely low-grade, but it's there 90 per cent of the time. Maybe once in three months I can get up and feel energy, and it might last for a day or two if I'm lucky, then I'm back to my normal standard.

I can't imagine somebody getting up every day being bright and bubbly, and ready to go.

It's still there at a level below what I'm coping with. I'm scared of totally crashing when it gets out of my control, and I've got professionals stepping in and telling me what I need to do. I want to do it my way.

I'm not very proactive. I can understand it in my head, but I'm not very good at taking the next step and having to work at it. I've found my little niche now, where at least I'm still going out to work, still being independent.

For me, it's the simple things, I think, that seem to be very effective. When you're really down, you find that you look back and find that you drag yourself along, you really have to just push yourself. Move faster, lift your head up, move even at a brisker pace. I've got a skirt, a wraparound skirt, one of those old-fashioned ones, it's a full-length one. And that's my way of feeling special. I can wear that around the house, and I can feel a little bit feminine.

I've been on my own for a good 10 to 15 years, and that's what I need because there's nobody else's standards I feel like I've got to keep up with. People have asked me why I don't move into town, but for me, trying to cope with high rents, dealing with a scary landlord and having to match up to somebody's standards all the time, I just feel like I don't fit. That's why it's easier for me to stay at home, be a homebody. That's where I'm safe.

A couple of summers ago, my son and I actually painted the outside of our house. (Part of managing depression) is knowing when you can push yourself. Other days you can get all geared up to go out there with a steel brush and start sanding, and you just look at the wall and go: "Nope. Not today."

It's just learning that some days you need a kick in the butt. You can say: "Right, I'm gonna get the dishes done." Other days, no kick in the butt's going to get you moving. So those days, it's okay, just sit. If all you do today is breathe, that's fine. You've achieved something. You've just got to break it down to the smallest steps. Not even getting through an hour of the day. Sometimes, it's just going through minute-by-minute.

Chapter Sixteen: Michelle

It was two o'clock in the morning, and I was sitting out on the deck with a coffee and cigarette, in a dark, depressive state. I'd been thinking of all the ways I could commit suicide. How I could do it, where I would do it.

It even crossed my mind that I couldn't do it at home because there would be too many people coming and going from the household at different times, with some working different shifts and what have you. I would have to go somewhere off-site, I thought.

This wasn't me. This felt like it was somebody else's conversation, not my own. These were not my thoughts. My head was trying to stop these thoughts and it was like I was trying to fight my own mind.

"This is wrong," I said to myself. "I shouldn't be thinking like this. I don't want to think like this."

But the thoughts were still there. No matter how much I tried to get them out of my head, I couldn't.

Then my son came home. He'd been out with his friends. He made himself a coffee and came to sit out with me on the deck. He began telling me all about his night out.

I got up, said goodnight and went to bed. The next morning, I told my husband what had happened and what I'd been thinking, so we sought help from the mental health team.

I'd had depression from my teens, I think. I didn't know what it was back then, but I had all the symptoms. Being very lethargic, having no enthusiasm, loss of motivation, sleep disturbances, all those sorts of things that come with depression, but obviously not to the point where I was in any danger of hurting myself; just being really, really sad for long periods of time. I was never put on any medication. Not then.

After I had my two sons, I had a breakdown. My GP put it down to post-natal depression being previously undiagnosed and prescribed anti-depressants and sleeping tablets. I stayed on that medication on and off for a few years, but everything seemed to be okay.

Obviously, there are things that happen in the course of your life, like the death of a loved one; certain events that bring you down to a sad state, but nothing that would cause you to self-harm without there being some sort of underlying problem. It's all part of living, grieving; all part of life.

Then it all blew up.

I'd had a goitre (a swelling in the neck resulting from an enlarged thyroid gland) on the left side of my neck for about three years. My doctor didn't appear to be in any hurry to do anything about it, obviously because I was coping. Then one day, I went to the doctor as it had been starting to get bigger in size.

It wasn't my normal doctor; it was a locum.

I said: "Look, I am actually getting quite concerned about this lump in the side of my neck. It seems to be growing, and I've had it for quite some time."

He got on the computer and looked at the history.

"Yes, you've had it for three years. Why was nothing done?"

"I don't know," I said.

So he got out his camera, took photos and sent them through to the specialist, then sent me for blood tests. Sometime later, I got a phone call from the hospital, and they removed the left side (of my thyroid). Three months later was my first experience with being suicidal.

My bloodwork had apparently been borderline normal, so they figured I had no need for medication.

I talked to a retired nurse, and she had told me that it happens quite a bit with the removal of the thyroid. I haven't done any research on it, but she told me that the T3 and T4 hormones, if they are just at that normal level, there is a tendency to end up being suicidal afterwards.

After that night and those suicidal thoughts, I was admitted to the mental health unit. I volunteered to stay for a week. There I was assessed and told I was showing the majority of signs that I had bipolar (otherwise known as manic depression). I was put on medication for mood stabilising, anti-psychotics, and sleeping tablets to try and calm me down and bring me back to some sort of level.

I went home, had a couple of weeks off work, felt a lot better, went back to work, and life carried on as normal.

Every couple of weeks, I would get a phone call from my case nurse just to check on me and see how I was doing. Every three months, I would see the psychologist to review my case and monitor my moods to see whether I was manic or depressive and how many little depressive outbursts I'd had.

I was put on some type of sedative type medication which left me feeling very very drugged, to the point where I couldn't perform my job, so I was given amitriptyline to counteract the drugginess the next day.

Within three weeks of taking that, I spiralled down back into a suicidal state.

This time it was different. This time I wanted to physically hurt myself. I knew those thoughts were there, and I was trying to fight them and stop them, but it was definitely thoughts toward hurting myself that time.

I spent another week at the respite, and I was taken off almost all medication.

In the process, I lost my job.

I am still not working, and I am only just starting to get over the feeling of being overwhelmed, terrified of going back into the workplace. I am looking at options, what I want to do, when I return back to the workforce. I'm even considering doing some study instead, although I don't know how to go about it at this stage.

The whole thing has been hard on my family. My two boys reacted differently, as people do. My older one just sort of withdrew and shut down, got very, very quiet, got very angry at me. My younger son sort of understood because he's had bouts of depression himself. He was actually very supportive and very caring.

My husband got counselling. Every now and again he'll still get a phone call from the counselling people to find out how he's doing. It was explained to him what bipolar is, how it will affect me, what to expect in mood swings and changes, that sort of thing. So, he now has an understanding of why I do the strange, quirky things that I do that I'm not aware that I'm doing. He'll just sort of think, oh, here we go, let's just step back and let her go, let her have her rant and her silly whatever.

It's tiring for him because it's like it's on this loop, round and round. We do have a bit of a not so much an argument, more a frustrated conversation about my mental health, and how I get stuck in these low moods and I can't seem to get out of them. I'm in these low moods for … it could be days, it could be weeks and there's no telling how long and he just turned around and said: "I am tired of being the carer for your mental health."

Because it is hard. Hard for those on the outside. Sometimes, I think harder than me dealing with it, because half the time I'm oblivious to what I do, what I say. I've lost friends because of things that have happened, things that I've said, because I'm in one of my angry moods or whatever.

There is guilt - for putting your family and your friends through so much pain. You feel guilt for doing the things you do, saying the things you say; the lack of motivation, the lack of zest for life that you should have just to do the normal things.

I've had about four different psychologists in the course of a year and they all have varied opinions. Two of them prescribed minimal drugs but natural remedies; things like working on your mindfulness and diet and exercise - natural ways of coping. I've had one that just drugged me up to the eyeballs with everything possible and treat the symptoms that way.

I prefer to manage it with minimal drugs and using the natural, holistic way with mindfulness, meditation, eliminating the stresses in your life, diet and exercise. I always feel better when I've been for a walk. Putting the music on the headphones and off you go. You don't actually realise how far you've walked when you're just focusing on getting your head in the right space. Quite often, I can go between six to 10 kilometres just in a circuit around town.

I prefer doing that rather than being drugged up and oblivious to what's going on around me because of the medication.

I hate the thought of being medicated. Even in the past with having the anti-depressants, I just hated the thought of taking this tablet so I could function. I thought there's got to be some other way. Like, why can I not function without having this tablet numbing me?

When you're drugged, your senses are dulled as well. You don't experience things like you do when you're not medicating. You're in this fog. It's like there's something missing all the time. Everything you do, you've got this feeling that there's something missing, something not right. You should be experiencing more. You should be feeling a lot more. Like going outside and walking on the grass in bare feet. Being with nature, the birds, breeze on your face, the sun. When you're drugged, I don't think you get that full experience; you don't feel, you don't smell, you don't hear. It's just everything's numbed. You're not living it. I hate that feeling.

I would like to think that at some stage, someday, I could be unmedicated.

I know that some of the medications that I had been put on –

some of the side effects are enhanced anxiety and suicidal thoughts, and I'm thinking: why are you prescribing this medication to someone who has the inclination to head in that direction to start with? Why? It doesn't make sense.

Some of the side effects, I think, make the problem worse. I felt worse when I came out of my second bout because I was on such a cocktail of drugs and some of those drugs were just to counteract side effects. Why not eliminate the drug that was causing the side effect? Rather than prescribe another one to counter and then another one to counteract that side effect. So, instead of being on one tablet you end up on five, because you've got side effects and you're being prescribed more to counteract those side effects. Is it necessary to be on five tablets? I just think that sometimes our doctors just like to write the prescriptions too much.

I believe in talking about it. I feel the more you talk about it, the more the brain can process it. I talk about it all the time.

I think the more we talk about it, the more people are made aware of it. Just to dispel that stigma. It can happen to anyone at any time. There is no discrimination. Like (2018), there were so many celebrities - it was shocking. You wouldn't have thought it of those people because of their public personas.

I suppose we all have our faces that we put on to hide it. I know I did. Because in my work (in retail), you have to smile and say hello and be extremely welcoming. As much as you're not feeling it, you put on a show.

People don't realise that when you have been suicidal, and you have been in that dark, deep place, it does change you. I've had a lot of comments from friends: "Oh, you've changed. You're not the same."

Of course I'm not going to be the same. I've had it twice in a 12-month period. I've wanted to, haven't physically attempted but the thought pattern was to end my life. Of course it's going to leave some sort of scar. It's going to change your thinking. It's got to. You can't just snap out of it and be the same person.

It does change you. It's hard to explain how, but you feel things differently too. More intense, I think.

I've become very cynical. I don't allow people to be disrespectful in any way, whether it's their tone of voice, what they say, their body language, or whatever. If it's directed at me, I shut it down. I won't let it go. I actually deal with it then and there.

I've become that person where it's: "Excuse me, you have no right to talk to me like that. It's not my fault you're angry." That sort of thing. In retail, you have to do that. You have to allow that angry customer to come in with a complaint and shout and scream and you have to sort of stand there and smile and say: "Oh, I'm so sorry, but let me try and fix this for you," in a nice manner, when these people are being downright rude. And it's not your fault.

Now, I won't put up with that. If somebody comes and starts at me, I'm like: "Hang on a minute. You have no right to talk to me like this. It's not acceptable. I'm not going to allow you to do it. This is your problem, your attitude problem, not mine."

I've become more self-protective, emotionally. I suppose now the guards are up all the time. I'm sort of in my little bubble and anybody who tries to be disrespectful, I retaliate.

I can see the funny side of it as well. I can laugh at myself. The silly things I do and say. I say it how it is - no filters, no boundaries.

I get very passionate about things to the point where it's an assertiveness. It's an: "I am here, I am me, accept it. This is it. This is who I am now. I wasn't this person before but this is me now and you either accept that or you don't."

Chapter Seventeen: Lucy

It all started when I began to lose interest in my boyfriend. We'd been together a while, but I just lost interest in anything to do with him. I began to notice a loss of pleasure in a lot of things, and I started self-harming. My best friend was unwell, both medically and mentally and was in hospital, and I was crying all the time. I think that may have been one of the things that triggered it all.

I was 17, going on 18. My school counsellor, who I'd been meeting with, wrote a letter to my GP, telling him I was showing symptoms of depression. That visit to the GP was not a good experience. He hummed and hahed and said: "Oh, maybe it's this," suggesting I had low iron. A blood test refuted that.

He prescribed anti-depressants for me, but didn't really give me any kind of education about it. He never even came out and said: "You've got depression." It was all really kind of 'hush-hush'.

He'd been my family GP for years, but I felt that he wasn't very good at dealing with mental health issues. It was frustrating. I just wanted to know what was wrong with me, so I could fix it. I eventually ended up changing GPs.

My mother's reaction was not positive. She had gone with me to the doctor, worried that I was crying all the time. I felt like shit, and I just didn't know why.

Mum was not so understanding at first. "We don't do depression in this family," she would say. "Just get on with it, get over it. Be positive."

The anti-depressants didn't help. Nothing really changed for me, and I ended up self-harming quite badly all the time. This got me referred to the adolescent mental health service. That was not a good experience either.

The doctor there was not helpful, especially with his attitude toward my depression and my self-harming.

"You're bored with your life," he would tell me. "You just need a hobby."

I was prescribed different anti-depressants, but again, didn't find my time in the service very helpful, so I ended up self-discharging.

I left home and began seeing an independent psychologist for cognitive behaviour therapy. I learnt a lot about unhelpful thinking styles. Things like how I thought wasn't very helpful sometimes and black-and-white thinking. Other things like catastrophising. The problem was, I never felt like the root of my depression was ever explored. I didn't even know what it was.

I saw the psychologist for about three years and felt I did make a little progress. I even went off the medication. However, in my second year of seeing her, I was going in and out of depressive episodes, and at the same time, I developed an eating disorder.

She was amazing and very supportive. We did get along very well, and she did help with a few things, but it didn't solve the problem.

I decided to start studying a course in the health field. It was something I wanted to do to help people. It probably sounds a bit cliched, but since I'd had such a bad experience with the health service myself, I didn't want other people to go through that same experience. I thought if I could change that for one person, that would be a good thing. I do feel that I have that emotional intelligence and awareness of my own condition to be able to use that experience to help others.

I did really well in my course, despite the fact that I had to come out a couple of times due to being unwell. I completed it and got a job in my chosen field.

I managed to stay in the role for a few months before I had another depressive episode, combined with a relapse of my eating disorder, and because of it, I lost my job.

I'd gone off my medication, thinking I didn't need it, and I felt a bit upset with myself over that. A lot of people had said to me when I had the relapse, that if I didn't get back on my medication I would lose my job. I just thought I'd be all right. That wasn't the case.

I didn't want to believe that I needed it. I went through this phase of saying that all I needed was therapy. That that would rewire my brain, and then I wouldn't have to take medication. I wanted to fix it myself, but I was in denial. I wanted to believe that I didn't need it. Maybe I saw that as a personal failure even though I don't think the same of other people who take it. To me, it was just that I failed because I couldn't fix my own depression.

After I lost my job, I spent several months in treatment, and I'm back on my medication. I know now that I have to take it if I want to get back into my chosen career.

It was difficult at the beginning with my family. Especially with some of my extended family. Some of them would just tell me to be positive, thinking that I just needed to do certain things to fix it. They'd say something like: "You just need to be busy. You need a routine. You need to go back to work, or study." Yes, it does help me, but it doesn't cure me.

Now they're more understanding and realise that I don't choose to be a downer, so they're really supportive. It's taken a few years, but they understand.

I have things I do to manage it. I go walking every morning, and I listen to music and motivating podcasts. I go to therapy - the psychologist I have now is really good.

I take my medication and try to eat healthily. I don't drink alcohol because that's a depressant and spend time with my pets.

Animals are great therapy.

I've got a good group of friends now who are understanding and supportive. For instance, if we're meant to hang out and I'm not having a good day, I just tell them how I'm feeling, and they understand.

Talking with friends helps, depending on who I'm with. It gets you out of your head a little bit. It's so easy to ruminate. I tend to isolate myself, so usually what I need is just to be around someone, even if it's not doing anything.

For the future, I would like to go back to work. I'd also like to travel some day. I try not to think too far ahead, though. Just get through the next couple of months.

The only advice I can give to someone who suspects they have depression is that I think it's important that if you go to a doctor and they don't listen, go to another doctor or keep trying to get them to listen. The same with therapy. If you can't find the right one, don't give up and just try to find someone who gets it.

Section Three
Famous People with Depression or Mental Illness

One of the biggest problems with depression is the lack of understanding. Especially for those who would apparently have no reason to be depressed.

There are various famous people still alive today who have openly discussed their own battles with depression. These people are successful actors, writers, musicians, business people and in some cases, multi-millionaires. Yet they often say that they have come across prejudice and ignorance. There are some who, without thinking, ask why that person is so unhappy when they are so successful.

The general consensus is that depression is debilitating. However, it must be noted that not all depressive episodes can be so debilitating that the sufferer is physically incapable of carrying out any semblance of a normal life. This bears repeating: the fact that a person shows themselves as capable of carrying out normal day-to-day tasks does not imply an absence of depression. The mere act of focusing on what is needed to be done may sometimes be the catalyst for holding such symptoms at bay.

As we have already learned from the deaths in recent years of some well-known (and some not so well-known in certain circles) people, that the fact they have made a success of their lives is completely irrelevant when it comes to depression.

Some figures in history have also been known to have had some form of mental illness, not least of which is depression. Some historians may debate this, but where possible, I will let the facts speak for themselves.

Biographical information has been sourced through research by reading biographies, Wikipedia and various magazine and newspaper articles. With thanks to the *New York Times*, especially. Biographies are referenced in the bibliography merely as books for further reading.

Wikipedia has been used for basic facts, but please note that complete accuracy of these facts cannot be guaranteed.

Chapter Eighteen: Winston Churchill

Sir Winston Leonard Spencer-Churchill was a British politician, statesman, writer and army officer. He was twice Prime Minister of Britain - his first time in office was at the height of the Second World War.

Born into an aristocratic family on the 30th of November, 1874, his childhood was apparently a difficult one, according to some biographies. His parents, Lord Randolph Churchill and Jennie (nee Jerome) have been described as 'distant'.

He did not do well in school. At seven, he was sent to boarding school and tended to 'act up'. As he grew older, his grades improved, but his behaviour did not (Wikipedia). Various stories recalled he was unhappy at school and along with bouts of ill health, it meant he lagged behind his classmates.

He was accepted to a military academy, after at least two attempts and served in the British Army for some years before entering politics.

Churchill married his wife Clementine (nee Hozier) in 1908. The couple were married for 57 years and had five children. Their second youngest daughter, Marigold, died of sepsis before she was three. Their eldest daughter, Diana, died in 1963. Her death was ruled a suicide.

In some biographies, mention has been made of a 'Black Dog', and most historians feel this referred to depression. Certainly, there seemed to be episodes in his life where he was depressed.

However, there is considerable debate among those in the field of psychology who do not see these as being indicative of having depression.

It is certain that events such as his daughter's death would have been the source of much grief. Churchill did suffer some financial loss as a result of the Wall Street Crash and of course, he was prime minister during much of World War Two.

He was also in a serious accident in 1931 which led to a period of low moods.

In a post on the website for the International Churchill Society, therapist and university professor Carol Breckenridge refuted claims that he suffered from manic depression.

She noted that his restlessness and periods of misbehaviour in school were characteristic of attention deficit disorder (Breckenridge, 2012).

Another suggested that his hyperactivity, irritability and mood swings were symptoms of depression. There were some members of his family who apparently did suffer from it (Ghaemi, 2012).

Without a comprehensive analysis of Churchill's life, however, it is difficult to say who is right.

Churchill died from a stroke on the 24th of January, 1965. He was 90.

He wrote several books, including memoirs, and one novel.

Chapter Nineteen: Isaac Newton

Known as the man who discovered gravity, mathematician and scientist Isaac Newton was born on December 25, 1642, although some biographies state he was born a few days later. This may be due to different calendars – one being the Julian and the other being the Gregorian - being used at the time.

His father, also Isaac Newton, had died a few months before. According to research, it appears the baby was premature. He was a sickly child and small for his age (Wikipedia).

His mother remarried and he was left in the care of his grandparents at the family home of Woolsthorpe Manor, in a hamlet in Lincolnshire, slightly more than 150 kms from London. The manor is now held by a trust and people visit to learn more about the scientist and his discoveries.

His mother's marriage may have caused some resentment as there are suggestions he kept some kind of list of 'sins' and one entry he wrote threatened harm to his mother and stepfather.

He began his education at The King's School in Grantham, Lincolnshire, England. The school website notes it as "Isaac Newton's School". In its history it states he attended the school from 1655 to 1660. His signature is allegedly written on a wall in one of the old buildings although it is unconfirmed as his (King's School history).

When he was seventeen, his mother tried to force him to return home to the manor to become a farmer. Instead, his teacher persuaded her to allow him to return to school.

In 1661, he began studying at Trinity College in Cambridge, completing a BA in 1665. The school was closed due to a plague epidemic which lasted about 18 months and killed an estimated 100,000 people (Wikipedia). It was the second plague in the span of 400 years (the first pandemic was in the 14th century).

Newton returned to Woolsthorpe where it is said he developed his theories on optics, calculus, and of course, gravity.

There are various theories around whether Newton had some kind of mental illness. His manner was described as distant. Research suggests this started in childhood, firstly with his mother's marriage, then refusal to play with other children.

He would have periods of insomnia, staying up late into the night. He also ate little.

His temper was apparently volatile in that he would often fight with peers, particularly over his theories, replying to any criticism with resentment.

Whether he truly had mental illness is still a subject of debate.

Newton never married and was close to very few people. He died on the 20th of March, 1727, at the age of 85.

Chapter Twenty: Charles Darwin

Charles Darwin is considered the founder of evolutionary theory and is most famous for his work: *On the Origin of Species,* as well as *The Descent of Man.*

For many years, Darwin was plagued by mysterious chronic illnesses that researchers have attempted to explain. Given these conditions and the length of time he suffered from them, it is very likely he had depressive episodes, as documented through letters sent to his family.

Born on the 12th of February 1809, in Shopshire, England, the second-last of six children. His mother Susannah (nee Wedgewood) died when he was eight.

His father, Robert Waring Darwin was a medical doctor. He would attempt to follow in his father's footsteps, enrolling at Edinburgh University to study medicine. However, it was in natural history that he found his niche.

When he showed no interest in medicine, he was sent to study at Christ's College in Cambridge. According to the college's website, the school included several eminent scholars who "sought to harmonise traditional Christian faith with the new truths of natural science" (Christ's College History). This was where Darwin's interest in botany and geology began.

While there, he began experiencing ill health, starting with mouth sores and eczema.

He finished his Bachelor's Degree, leaving Cambridge in June

1831. In August of that year, he was offered the opportunity to travel on an expedition to chart the coast of South America on the HMS Beagle.

While waiting to join the ship, he began complaining of chest pain and heart palpitations. However, he told no one and would only later admit to it in his autobiography (Campbell & Matthews, 2015).

On that voyage, he kept a diary of the things he learnt, which would later form the basis of his research.

He wrote of suffering various ailments including seasickness, exhaustion and loss of appetite.

In 1835, the ship visited the Galapagos Islands, an archipelago of volcanic islands in the Pacific Ocean and part of the Republic of Ecuador. Darwin would observe various bird species and those observations would lead him to his theories of natural selection and evolution.

His chronic health problems were put down to strain from working on his journal and his research and he was told to take some time off. He went to stay with relatives in the country, where he met his cousin, Emma Wedgwood. The couple married in 1839.

There were times when he would fail to turn up to events, which some researchers thought was out of a fear to face his critics. However, it could also be explained as an anxiety disorder.

Some researchers suggested that his illness was caused by nervous stress, brought on by the strain of his work, as well as some personal losses. His second child, daughter Annie, died at the age of ten.

An article in the Biological Journal of the Linnean Society states that Darwin had a chronic illness lasting 40 years. "Over 40 causes have been proposed to explain his illness. They fall into two main categories – psychosomatic and organic. Psychosomatic causes include bereavement syndrome, hyperventilation and panic attack, and depression." (Campbell & Matthews, 2015. Used with author's permission)

Darwin would write of his struggles to a friend. "I had a terrible long fit of vomiting yesterday, which makes the world rather extra gloomy today."

Campbell and Matthews note that the effect of his ill health is evident in letters written to family. The authors add that the proposed causes could match up to some of the symptoms, but not all.

The article states that Darwin tried a range of therapies, including some which would now be considered poisons, for example arsenic and bismuth. "Darwin's father ... recommended logwood, from the tree Haematoxylum campechianum, used to treat chronic diarrhoea, dysentery and haemorrhages from uterus, lungs or bowels."

The authors state their belief that Darwin was suffering from lactose intolerance. There are theories that there is a correlation between gut health and mental health.

Incidentally, in a communication with Professor Campbell, he told me that while lecturing in 2014, he met the great, great, great granddaughter of Charles Darwin who informed him that she was lactose intolerant.

Modern-day medicine confirms there is a link between chronic illness and depression and it is likely that Darwin's depression stemmed from his suffering various ailments over the four decades. Professor Campbell also posits this theory.

Darwin's research was published in volumes such as: On the Origin of Species (1859), The Descent of Man (1871) and several others.

He died at the age of 73 on the 19th of April, 1882.

Chapter Twenty-One: Abraham Lincoln

Abraham Lincoln was an American lawyer and politician who became the 16th President of the United States. He is also known as the President who passed the Emancipation Proclamation, which abolished slavery during the Civil War, although it would not truly be abolished until the ratification of the 13th Amendment to the U.S. Constitution in 1865.

Lincoln was born into a poor family in Kentucky, on the 12th of February, 1809. The family moved to Indiana when he was seven. Two years later, his mother, Nancy (nee Hanks) died. His sister, who was two years older than him, was left in charge until his father remarried a year later. Sarah Lincoln would die in childbirth ten years later (Wikipedia).

Research suggests that Lincoln's father preferred him to work on the farm, while the young Abraham preferred reading. His father was apparently very critical of his laziness. Given that Thomas Lincoln, according to research, was illiterate, he probably placed more importance on working the land than in an education.

When he was 21, Lincoln and his family moved to Illinois. He invested in a business but soon gave that up for politics, running unsuccessfully for the Illinois General Assembly before serving four terms in the state House of Representatives.

He became a lawyer and practiced for several years until becoming President. He was very vocal about his opposition to slavery - a policy that would later lead to the Emancipation Proclamation during the Civil War.

Some sources say he had a relationship with a woman named Ann Rutledge, which ended with her death. He became engaged to Mary Todd, whose parents were slaveowners, in 1840. The engagement was called off in 1841 for reasons which were never stated. The couple married in 1842 and would go on to have four sons together. All but one died before they reached adulthood.

Lincoln was known for being broody and a deep melancholy, which is now known as clinical depression.

An article in *The Atlantic* stated he was known for reciting poetry that was often gloomy. Although he was known for his humour, friends and acquaintances recalled he would talk of suicide (Shenk, 2005).

Lincoln was also apparently known for anxiety. Some research mentions hypochondria. Modern definition states this to be a condition in which a person is excessively and unduly worried about having a serious illness. It is now classed as a 'somatic symptom disorder' where a person feels extreme anxiety. The definition may have differed in Lincoln's time, but the connection is there.

Some researchers suggest that much of his depression stemmed from the losses in his youth, such as the deaths of his mother and his sister.

He carried on despite his melancholy. As some suggest, it was not in him to just give in to the depression (Ability Magazine).

He was elected to the presidency in 1860, leading a divided country through the Civil War. In 1863, he used his presidential powers to make the Emancipation Proclamation, freeing slaves in the southern states which had broken away from the union over the slavery issue. The proclamation was considered a measure of wartime and it was not until 1864 that a proposed amendment to the Constitution was read in Congress and passed in the House in January of 1865. It was officially ratified in December of that year, a move that Lincoln never lived long enough to see.

He was shot at Ford's Theatre in Washington on April 14, 1865 by John Wilkes Booth. He died the next morning.

Chapter Twenty-Two: Samuel Clemens

Samuel Clemens, who was better known as author Mark Twain, was a famous writer of several books including *The Adventures of Tom Sawyer, The Adventures of Huckleberry Finn, A Connecticut Yankee in King Arthur's Court, Life on the Mississippi* and several others.

Born Samuel Langhorne Clemens on November 30, 1835, his family lived in Florida, Missouri until he was four years old.

Clemens had six siblings but only three would make it to adulthood. His father, John, was an attorney, who died when Clemens was 11-years-old. By then, the family was living in Hannibal, Missouri, which would later be the inspiration for the setting of his books *The Adventures of Tom Sawyer* and *The Adventures of Huckleberry Finn*.

He left school at 12 to work in the printing trade, but then became a steamboat pilot.

His autobiography talks in detail of the death of his brother Henry, at just 20. According to research, including Wikipedia, Henry began working on a steamboat as a Mud Clerk. This essentially was someone who assisted in most of the roles aboard the boats. In May of 1858, Henry was mortally wounded when the boiler exploded. Clemens had claimed to have dreamed about the incident prior to it happening (Wikipedia). He apparently felt so guilty that he blamed himself for it.

Clemens married Olivia Langdon in 1870. The couple had a

son and three daughters: Susy, Clara and Jean. Their son, Langdon, died before he was two. Susy would pass away in 1896.

Clemens was also a public speaker, undertaking engagements in a world tour which included Australia, New Zealand, Fiji, and India, to name a few.

He also spent a few years in Europe, primarily in England.

There were financial struggles, firstly in childhood, after his father's death, then later in life when he lost money on a number of bad investments. These, as well as his personal tragedies, contributed to his negative thoughts and feelings. An article on historyaccess.com states he also began to suffer geriatric depression – this was not well-known in the first decade of the twentieth century (Frost, 2002).

Clemens' autobiography also mentioned depression but he chose to focus on his work.

He was also famous for saying that he was born with Halley's Comet and would go out with it. His words proved to be prophetic. He died of a heart attack on 21 April, 1910, one day after the comet passed close to Earth. He was 74.

Chapter Twenty-Three: Tennessee Williams

Famed playwright Tennessee Williams was born Thomas Lanier Williams in the city of Columbus, Mississippi in 1911. He was the second child of Edwina Dakin and Cornelius Williams. Cornelius was a travelling salesman. Research suggests Williams' father was abusive, although it is unclear how abusive.

Williams would later recall that the marriage between his parents was difficult (*New York Times*, 1983). However, not long after the family moved to St Louis, a third child was born – Walter Dakin Williams.

Biographers state he was close to his older sister, who would later experience psychotic episodes. Williams himself believed he had borderline psychosis, as mentioned in an obituary, but was able to turn that psychosis into his writing.

Plagued by ill-health as a child, he made up stories to keep himself and his sister occupied, although some suggest this led to him becoming rather introverted. Certainly, friends would later recall that he was rather a shy or timid man (Kakutani, 1983).

The family apparently moved a few times, which would later be reflected in Williams' own restlessness.

At the age of eighteen, Williams enrolled at the University of Missouri to study journalism, but later dropped out and got a job at a shoe factory. It was at this point that he began to show signs of depression that would be a constant throughout the rest of his life.

To combat his feelings, he would write stories and poetry, often staying up late. Following a nervous breakdown, he again enrolled at university in 1937. He graduated from the University of Iowa in 1938. He had already written several plays, and some were produced on campus.

By this time, Rose's psychotic episodes had become out of control and the family decided to allow an experimental procedure to be performed – a prefrontal lobotomy. Sadly, while it did help calm her, it also left her in a state where her memory was badly affected. She spent the rest of her life in a sanatorium.

Williams moved to New Orleans, changing his first name to Tennessee. His reason for doing so was unclear. Some speculated that he had chosen that name as he had spent time with his beloved grandparents in Tennessee. Others thought it was a nickname.

His experiences became part of the backdrop to one of his most famous plays, *A Streetcar Named Desire.*

His plays, especially *Streetcar* and *Glass Menagerie* seemed to draw on some of his own experiences, and probably his own struggles with mental health. Some of his characters would have parallels with some of his family.

He once said his interest was more in creating characters who were flawed in some way. "I suppose I have found it easier to identify with the characters who … were frightened of life, who were desperate to reach out to another person."

In spite of his troubles, he continued to work at his writing.

Friends and admirers would later remark on his tenacity. Theatre director and producer Josè Quintero was quoted in an article in the New York Times. "Whenever I despaired of my own work, I thought of his courage in the face of so much pain." (Kakutani, 1983).

His shyness was another issue. Some friends would comment that he was not good at expressing himself verbally, often saying things that could be misunderstood. In his writing, however, it appeared easier.

Williams' last few years were marked by failures. His plays were panned by critics and did not perform well. Famed writer and director Elia Kazan told the *New York Times* that Williams carried on anyway, although it deeply affected him.

"It left a hole in him, and the melancholy grew over him in those last years."

The death of his former partner and reliance on drugs and alcohol were major contributors in the decline in his mental health. Williams had lived with Frank Merlo for some years and although they were no longer lovers at the time of Merlo's death in 1963, it still grieved him.

He feared his mortality. Some reported that he would always say he wasn't well and thought he was dying, although they did not go so far as saying he was a hypochondriac.

Williams struggled with alcoholism and drugs. His brother, Dakin, told a Times reporter that he had Williams confined to a hospital in St Louis in 1969 (Gussow, 1983). Research suggests that this confinement led to a period of estrangement between the siblings.

Tennessee Williams died in February 1983, at the age of 71. Initial reports were that it was 'natural causes' but an autopsy revealed he died from asphyxiation after choking on a bottle cap.

The playwright was a prolific writer, leaving behind a huge legacy which many writers who were born after him aspired to. He wrote 38 plays – all but nine were major plays, and several were adapted into movies or teleplays. He also wrote two novels, several short stories, poems, and one-act plays (Wikipedia).

Chapter Twenty-Four: Judy Garland

Judy Garland achieved much in her short life, but to some, the one thing that was out of reach for this incredibly talented singer and actress was happiness.

In a special report in the New York Times, after she was found dead in her London home at the age of 47, it was written that her life seemed to be a "fruitless search for the happiness promised in *Over the Rainbow*."(*New York Times*, 1969) The song from the movie that made her famous was full of lines about dreams of troubles melting away.

She later said it was symbolic of her own dreams and wishes.

Had she been able to melt those troubles away, perhaps her life would not have ended so prematurely.

Born Frances Ethel Gumm in Grand Rapids, Minnesota on the 10th of June, 1922, she was the youngest of three girls. Her parents, Frank and Ethel, had been involved in vaudeville.

The family moved to California in 1926.

All three girls were made to perform in shows, but it was clear early on who had the most talent, something which apparently caused some jealousy in her older sisters.

Garland's mother was, according to some sources, the epitome of the 'stage mother', forcing her youngest to practice instead of playing outside with friends like any normal child.

The girls performed in a variety of vaudeville shows, then short films.

In 1935, Garland was signed to Metro-Goldwyn-Mayer. At thirteen, she was too old to be a child star and too young for adult roles. Her looks were not considered glamorous, something which affected her self-esteem (Wikipedia).

Her father died later that year, another event which devastated the budding starlet. As reported in the *New York Times*, she wrote, many years later, that it had been "the most terrible thing that ever happened in my life". She went on to say that she hadn't had a close relationship with her father, although she wanted to – they had not really spent a lot of time together.

Her star grew, although it was hard work. She would often be teamed up with Mickey Rooney and the actors were good friends.

She had major confidence issues in which she was always unsure of herself.

What may not have helped was that when they were casting for *The Wizard of Oz* (1939), the studio originally wanted Shirley Temple. When she wasn't available, they wanted someone else. Garland was their third choice.

By the time filming began, she was sixteen years old. The character was supposed to be about twelve. She was forced to disguise her more adult figure.

The production itself was demanding on actors and crew alike. While other actors spoke well of Garland, they were less complimentary about the pressure put on them all.

At eighteen, she was already seeing a psychiatrist. She later wrote of her experience of telling her troubles to the man before going to the studio to work. At this point, she was taking stimulants and depressants – sleeping pills to knock her out and pep pills to wake her up, apparently given to her by the studio.

"That's the way we worked and that's the way we got thin. That's the way we got mixed up," she wrote (*New York Times*, 1969).

Garland began to gain a reputation for being difficult – something which would continue throughout her career, but part of it was more than likely due to the fact that the studio worked her extremely hard, barely giving her a chance to rest.

She married the first of her five husbands at age nineteen, divorcing him three years later.

One of Garland's most popular films was *Meet Me in St Louis (1944)*. She initially turned it down but eventually did agree to make the movie. Her time on set was not without its difficulties, especially the arguments between her and the director. What was most remarkable about this, however, was that the man who directed this film, Vincente Minnelli, became her second husband, and father of her daughter, Liza Minnelli. The couple divorced in 1951.

Garland was admitted to a sanatorium during this time – it was one of many admissions.

According to the *Times* obituary, she attempted suicide several times. Her third husband, Sid Luft, accused her of doing so at least 20 times. The couple had two children together.

Following her divorce from Minnelli, she performed solo shows in London and in New York, with great success, although it was noticeable that her voice was failing (*New York Times*, 1969).

She returned to Hollywood in 1954 to star in *A Star Is Born*, a remake of a film that first screened in the 1930s. Production was held up due to her erratic and apparently temperamental behaviour.

Garland's performance was praised, and she would go on to be nominated for an Oscar, but lost out to Grace Kelly.

She began performing in a weekly television show for CBS in 1963 but the show was only one season. She returned to performing on stage but that appeared to take its toll, both physically and mentally.

She married for the fourth time in 1965. This again ended in divorce. In 1969 she married Mickey Deans.

On the 22nd of June, 1969, she was found dead in the bathroom of her rented home. The coroner stated her cause of death was an overdose of barbiturates. It was ruled accidental.

Chapter Twenty-Five: Vincent van Gogh

If you have ever listened to the song *Vincent* (aka *Starry, Starry Night*) by Don McLean, you would probably know some of the history of Vincent van Gogh's life, as it tells a story of the artist's struggles with mental health and his eventual suicide.

McLean once wrote that he had been reading van Gogh's biography and felt the need to write something to defend the artist, especially against claims the man was crazy.

Most people who have heard of the Dutch artist think of him as a tortured soul who did not make a name for himself until after his death. There is the famous story of him cutting off his ear and sending it to a woman. Much of the story has been embellished in one way or another – that it was because of a rejection by a woman. A *New York Times* article (Gorman, 1923) mentions this story saying it was over some kind of joke at a brothel. Whether this story really happened or not is something we may never know, but it does suggest a man who was deeply troubled and struggled with mental health issues. At the very least, depression.

Vincent Willem van Gogh was born in Zundert, Netherlands in 1853. He was the eldest of six – two other boys and three girls. He remained close with one brother and one sister through his life (Wikipedia).

He would draw in his childhood but it wasn't until later in his short life that he began painting.

He took on a job as an art dealer, at first working The Hague before moving to London to work. After some troubles, he was sent to Paris. He lost his job and took on another role teaching in England.

He had a growing interest in religion, although research suggests it was more of an obsession. His behaviour and apparent restlessness in finding a role that suited him seem to be more signs that he was struggling with his mental health.

In 1880, he began studying at the <u>Académie Royale des Beaux-Arts</u>, a school for the arts in Belgium.

He would later be influenced by such artists as Paul Gauguin.

It is often said that there is a fine line between genius and madness, and van Gogh was probably the most well-known of that example (Robinson, 2011). More than a hundred years since his death, most psychologists are still at a loss to explain the artist's genius and madness both appearing to coexist.

Van Gogh is known as a post-impressionist painter who created hundreds of oil paintings in ten years. Sadly, his work went unrecognised during his life and he only became famous following his death.

He shot himself in the chest on the 27th of July 1890 and died two days later.

Chapter Twenty-Six: Calvin Coolidge

The 30th President of the United States, John Calvin Coolidge Jr was born in 1872 – the only President to be born on what is known as American Independence Day – on the 4th of July, in Plymouth, Vermont.

His mother, Victoria, died when he was twelve years old and his younger sister, Abbie, died five years later.

He would later write in his autobiography that Victoria's death was a life-changing moment for him.

Following his graduation from high school, he apprenticed to a lawyer in Massachusetts before being admitted to the bar (Wikipedia). He went on to open his own practice.

Coolidge met and later married Grace Anna Goodhue. The couple would have two sons, John and Calvin Jr.

His involvement in politics began with campaigning for Republican presidential candidate William McKinley in 1896, going on to serve on the Republican City Committee, the City Council of Northhampton, Massachusetts and clerk of courts.

In 1906, he was elected to the state House of Representatives where he would serve approximately three years before stepping down and returning to Northhampton and became mayor.

Coolidge ran for state senate, beginning his session in 1912 and winning re-election in 1913. It was apparently the custom to retire after two terms in the senate (terms being one year duration), however he decided to run again in 1914 and held the office of President of the Senate.

He was encouraged to run for lieutenant governor, an office he held from January 1916 to January 1919, where he took over office as governor of Massachusetts.

Coolidge was nominated as the Republican candidate for Vice-President alongside Warren G Harding for President in the 1920 Presidential elections. When Harding died unexpectedly in 1923, Coolidge became President.

Calvin Coolidge was known as a quiet man with a reputation for being stiff, but he would later write his own opinion that since everything he said as President was considered important, he needed to choose his words carefully.

In 1924, a devastating event would plunge the President into a deep depression. His youngest son, Calvin Jr, age sixteen, died from blood poisoning.

An article on a biography in *The Atlantic* magazine (Beatty, 2003) stated that Coolidge felt his son's death was akin to a punishment for his success. The man would later write in his autobiography that it was the 'price' for becoming President.

Coolidge showed several other characteristics of depressive disorder, including sleeping more. Much of the burden of his office went to his wife instead, while he avoided becoming involved in administrative decisions, among other things.

This certainly fits with some of the causes of depression. Given that he had most likely never really grieved for his mother or his sister, losing his younger son would have been the proverbial straw that broke him.

It was around this time that the economy began to show signs of collapse, leading to the Wall Street Crash in October 1929. Some historians blame the President's lack of action in regulating the excesses which led to the downturn. However, others argue that Coolidge considered commercial regulation, such as child labour laws and wage legislation, to be the role of state and local government, rather than federal government, as was apparently the custom in the 1920s.

Coolidge chose not to run again in the 1928 elections and stepped down as President, succeeded by Herbert Hoover.

The former President died in 1933.

Chapter Twenty-Seven: Others

Agatha Christie (1890 - 1976)

Born Agatha Miller on the 15th of September, 1890, she was known for her mystery novels featuring characters like Hercule Poirot and Miss Marple.

In 1926, the famed writer disappeared for 11 days. According to an article, her vehicle was found abandoned. Her fur coat and driver's licence were found inside.

Police launched a manhunt, but initially, it was assumed to be some sort of foul play. Christie's husband, Colonel Archibald Christie, had planned to divorce her for a young woman.

After those 11 days, Christie was found in a hotel under an assumed name and claimed amnesia.

However, it is not known if this amnesia was faked.

Some people believe Christie was depressed following the death of her mother. Others suggest she experienced depression due to stress from overwork or her husband's infidelity.

A writer used a theory about Christie's disappearance as the basis of a novel (Turner, 2017). The man claimed the truth was revealed in a semi-autobiographical novel in which the character apparently attempted suicide.

Christie died peacefully from natural causes on the 12th of January, 1976.

Virginia Woolf (1882-1941)

Born Adeline Virginia Stephen on the 25th of January, 1882, she was known for novels such as *To The Lighthouse* and *Mrs Dalloway*.

In a biographical analysis of Woolf on owlcation.com, the writer states the novelist was prone to nervous breakdowns and constantly lived in fear of these breakdowns.

Loss of family would have contributed to her mental health issues. When she was thirteen, her mother died. At fifteen, she lost a stepsister and a 'mother figure'. Then her father died in 1905.

While she was writing, her husband Leonard noticed she appeared well, but following the completion of a novel, she would be depressed (owlcation.com)

Information on Wikipedia states she had bipolar disorder. Although because much of her mental illness was mis-diagnosed it is difficult to say whether this was the correct diagnosis.

Woolf was institutionalised several times and attempted suicide. She died by suicide – she filled her pockets with stones and walked into the river near her home on the 28th of March, 1941.

Ernest Hemingway (1899-1961)

Born in Chicago on July 21, 1899, Ernest Miller Hemingway was a famous journalist and novelist. Following high school, he became a reporter in Kansas City.

Information available on *britannica.com* states he was an ambulance driver for the American Red Cross in World War I and at 18 was injured on the Austro-Italian front (Young, 2019).

He became a foreign correspondent post-war and published his first book, a collection of stories, in 1924.

He was known for several novels including: *The Sun Also Rises*, *The Old Man and the Sea*, *A Farewell to Arms* and *For Whom the Bell Tolls*, among others.

He received the Pulitzer prize in 1953 and the Nobel Prize for Literature in 1954.

An article on website National Post states Hemingway became an alcoholic. He would also struggle with depression, anger issues and paranoia, accusing others of trying to destroy him (Fulford, 2016).

He was hospitalised for mental health issues, both times at the Mayo Clinic in Minnesota.

He took his own life on July 2, 1961.

Marilyn Monroe

Actress Marilyn Monroe had a reputation for being difficult but she was considered a sex symbol in her time.

She was born Norma Jean Mortenson on 1 June, 1926. She was apparently illegitimate. Mortenson was the last name on her birth certificate. She later took her mother's last name of Baker.

There was mental illness in her family – her mother was committed to an asylum.

In an article in the New York Times, a studio chief was quoted as saying that she had felt she had some kind of psychological illness. She was also reported in a magazine article as saying she was "never used to being happy" (New York Times, 1962).

She married for the first time at sixteen, to an aircraft worker named James Dougherty. Her second marriage was to Yankees baseball player Joe DiMaggio. Her third to playwright Arthur Miller.

Her most famous films include: *The Seven-Year Itch* and *Some Like It Hot*.

She was found dead in her Los Angeles home on the 5th of August 1962. She was 36 years old. A bottle of that had contained sleeping pills was next to her bed.

Her death was ruled a suicide. However, some people still believe she was murdered.

Wolfgang Amadeus Mozart

The famous composer was born on the 27th of January, 1756 in Salzburg, Austria.

He was a child prodigy who began composing at around five years of age and composed more than 600 classical works.

Various websites claim he mentioned feeling depressed in letters sent to his family and a constant sadness – a symptom of major depressive disorder.

He died on the 5th of December, 1791 at the age of 35.

Herman Melville

Born on the 1st of August in 1819, in New York City, Herman Melville was most famous for the novel *Moby Dick*.

The novel included some of his own experiences working on a whaling ship.

Melville's father died when he was 13-years-old. The family struggled with poverty.

He had his own struggles with finances. While he wrote and published many short stories, he did not make a lot of money. Only a small number of copies of *Moby Dick* sold in his lifetime.

Many of his personal experiences found their way into his stories. In one of his short stories, a character had depression.

Melville died on the 28th of September, 1891 at the age of 72.

Hans Christian Andersen

Known as a writer of fairy tales such as *The Little Mermaid*, *The Ugly Duckling* and *The Snow Queen*, Andersen's had many struggles in his life.

He was born in Odense, Denmark on the 2nd of April, 1805.

When his father died in 1816, he was sent to a school for poor children and supported himself by working as an apprentice.

At 14, he moved to Copenhagen, to pursue dreams of working in the performing arts. He was encouraged to try writing.

He began studying at a school, but he was apparently abused and his teachers tried to discourage him from writing.

Andersen never married, although he had many infatuations with both men and women.

He died on the 4th of August, 1875, at the age of 70.

Raymond Chandler

Famous for creating the character of Philip Marlowe in *The Big Sleep*, Chandler was born on the 23rd of July, 1888 in Chicago.

His parents divorced and he moved with his mother to England when he was eight.

He tried working as a reporter, with not much success and served with the Canadian army in World War I.

He also worked in the oil industry but was struggling with his mental health and alcoholism.

His first novel was not published until 1939, although he had already published several short stories.

He married a woman 17 years older than him and was devastated when she died a few years before his own death. He again struggled with alcoholism and depression, also attempting suicide.

He died on the 26th of March, 1959. He was 70.

Section Four

Before we can even look at ways to manage depression, we need to understand it. I have researched several articles and texts to try to come up with a way to explain the illness itself.

Not everyone experiences depression the same way, and there are several theories around the illness.

Depression has been called many things over the years. Melancholia or Black Dog are just two of them. The term, according to an article cited in Wikipedia, was derived from the Latin verb deprimere, 'to press down' (Wikipedia).

The next chapter will look at how depression has been defined through history, and some of the ways it is defined and treated by the scientific and medical community, as well as society as a whole. I will attempt to debunk some of the myths about depression. Then I will look at some of the causes, both through research and my own experiences before ending this section with some statistics.

Ancient

According to an article on Wikipedia, personality types were thought to be determined by the dominant humour in a particular person - humour being thought to be basic bodily fluids. The Greeks considered disease to be an imbalance of these fluids. This may fit in with the school of thought that suggests depression is a chemical imbalance in neurotransmitters. However, not every expert agrees with this hypothesis. This will be explored later.

Hippocrates described melancholia, a word derived from the Ancient Greek melas (black) and kholé (bile) (Liddell & Scott (1980), as a distinct disease. He suggested symptoms were long-lasting fears and despondencies.

Hippocrates was writing around 400 BC, so the concept of melancholia is nothing new.

Around 5th Century BC, Greek playwright Sophocles produced a Tragedy known as *Ajax* (Sophocles, Translation Johnston, 2010). As is the case with many characters in Ancient Greek history and literature, the Romans created their own versions and Ajax was a Roman translation of the original name - the English transliteration of which is Aias.

In the play, after Achilles is killed in battle during the Trojan War, Ajax threatens to kill the two kings, Agamemnon and Menelaus after they give Achilles' armour to Odysseus. The Goddess Athena steps in and deludes Ajax into killing the spoil of the Greek army. When he comes to his senses, he realises what he has done and decides to commit suicide by impaling himself with his own sword.

There are hints of his depression in the following passage:

Aiai! My name is a lament!
Who would have thought it would fit
so well with my misfortunes!
Now truly I can cry out -- aiai! --
two and three times in my agony

What this illustrates quite clearly is that the concept of depression has been around for over two thousand years.

Black Dog

As a metaphor, the image of the Black Dog is a powerful way to describe depression. At its best, it's a dog that lolls about on the floor, refusing to get up to go for a walk. At its worst, it's the growling, snarling, teeth-bared, attack-mode dog that leaves you paralysed, wanting to run away and hide afraid it will find you and rip you to shreds.

The metaphor of the Black Dog in its contemporary form may be accredited to Winston Churchill, who directly referred to it in a letter to his wife in 1910. However, some writers debate that Churchill was meaning depression when he spoke about the Black Dog, although no alternative explanation is provided.

Eighteenth-century English writer, Samuel Johnson, was reported to have used it in a letter to a friend, according to an essay originally published on the website of the Black Dog Institute, although it is no longer available on that site. The letter referred to the friend's health.

Various mythologies have this image in common, depicting the black dog either as one of the Devil's guises, a witch's familiar, as guardian or gate-keeper of the world of the dead.

There are many myths that describe black dogs, like hellhounds, often assigned to guard the world of the dead. In

Greek mythology, this hound was known as Cerberus.

Some European folklore states that if someone stares into a hellhound's eyes three times, that person will die. J K Rowling, in her novel, *The Prisoner of Azkaban*, includes black dog imagery. Young wizard Harry Potter runs away from home and sees a black dog in the bushes. At school, he attends a class in Divination and when his professor sees the dog in tea leaves, she proclaims that it is The Grim, and he is about to die.

Generally, the appearance of the black dog is used as a harbinger of bad omen, which is more than likely why it has become almost synonymous with depression.

The term: Depression

By the 14th century, the word depression was seen to mean 'bring down in spirits' (Wikipedia, History of Depression) and slowly came into regular use. French psychiatrist Louis Delasiauve (1804-1893) used it in reference to a psychiatric symptom (Wikipedia). Melancholia (as discussed below) was still the dominant term used to diagnose the disorder, but it eventually was phased out, and depression became the more common term.

Freud

Sigmund Freud has, for much of the twentieth century, been considered the founder of psychoanalysis. His theories about dreams, the ego and the id, are the most well-known.

In 1917, Freud published an essay delving into the theories of melancholia. In the essay, he makes a clear distinction between mourning and melancholia.

However, he also cautioned against drawing any firm conclusions from his theories, stating that the definition of melancholia fluctuates. Whether this is the basis of current theories on depression or if other researchers have formed these warring theories independent of Freud is hard to say. Rather like the adage: 'which came first, the chicken or the egg'.

It suggests that there are different clinical illnesses which could be classified as melancholia, but cannot all be considered the same thing. Some of these were somatic, or relating to the body, while others could be psychological.

SO WHAT IS IT?

The Black Dog Institute in Australia states depression is a common medical condition. Statistics vary by country, but it is estimated that depression affects more than 300 million people around the world.

An article produced by the American National Institute of Mental Health includes data in which the parameters for major depressive episode included symptoms like the following:

- Periods of at least two weeks where someone is depressed or loses interest
- Problems sleeping, eating, lack of energy or concentration, poor self-image or recurrent thoughts of death or suicide.

Freud's definition goes into this in a little more detail. The list is taken from his writings but paraphrased.

- Low spirits to the point of emotional pain
- Lack of interest in the outside world
- Unable to love - what he means specifically by this is unclear
- Lack of motivation or interest in any activity
- Low self-esteem to the point of blaming yourself for the way things are, even hating yourself.

These match many of the feelings I have had over the years, especially the self-reviling. Even comedian Mike King, in a clip on TVNZ Current Affairs show Seven Sharp in March 2018, talked about the 'inner critic'. Psychology generally defines this as internal dialogue. It's often quite normal, however, with someone with depression, that voice is not only rather loud, but often tends to revisit past mistakes and berates oneself. It is often something like: "Why did you do that? You are so stupid!"

Is Depression A Disease?

We know depression is considered a medical condition. The question remains, how do we categorise it? Is it an illness, a disease or a mental condition?

Dr Stephen A. Diamond, Ph.D, posed this question in a post on his blog in *Psychology Today* (Diamond, 2008 – used with consent).

He questions the viability of applying what is known as the 'medical model' to the theory and practice of psychology and psychiatry. A clinical and forensic psychologist, he had worked in the field of psychotherapy for more than three decades at the time of posting.

"The medical model is the paradigm on which the practice of clinical medicine is founded: Symptoms are seen as manifestations of pathological physiological processes (disease) which are diagnosed and then treated with whatever methods available." (Diamond, 2008)

Basically, most diseases can be diagnosed and treated based on physiological symptoms or via pathological methods like blood tests, x-rays, or magnetic resonance imaging (MRI), for example.

To my knowledge, there is no such thing as a blood test, for example, to detect depression in a patient. So what Dr Diamond is suggesting to my mind is that the medical model as applied to mental illness is, at best, faulty, or to use his term, problematic.

Look on any depression website, like www.depression.org.nz, and you may find a self-test, but this in itself is not an accurate indicator of depression. For one thing, it relies on a patient's perception of how they are feeling. Not to say that this is inaccurate in itself, as diagnosis of any other illnesses also relies on this to some extent; however, problems can arise when a patient 'self-diagnoses'. While I do tend to research various symptoms before I decide to see my GP about something, I take it with a grain of salt and am careful not to make assumptions based on what I have read.

David Hill is a GP and director of the Health Hub Project in Palmerston North. In a chat with Dr Hill, I asked him how doctors diagnose depression. Generally, they have a guideline they have to follow, which in essence is much the same as the self-test in the above website.

GPs have various clinical resources, but unfortunately, much of these are limited, due to funding issues.

Dr Hill is a GP who is advocating for changes to the way PHOs (Primary Health Organisations) and district health boards in New Zealand administer the system, but it is one of those uphill battles that is yet to be resolved.

Dr Diamond also questions the treatment of depression under the medical model. Some people with depression can exhibit physical symptoms, like vomiting, diarrhoea, or insomnia - all of which I have experienced at one point or another. In the very worst cases, depression can lead to death by way of suicide.

Treatment depends on what the causes of the depression are. This is something on which many psychologists tend to disagree. This will be looked at further in the chapter on causes.

The question of whether depression is a disease is something that psychologists will also debate. The term disease implies that there is a standard treatment. Dr Diamond suggests that depression is not a disease in that sense, unlike diabetes or cancer, simply because there is no standardised treatment for it.

This is not to say that there are no physiological symptoms in some cases. Where the patient also has anxiety issues, these may present as physical symptoms, which may mask the psychosomatic ones.

In all cases, it is important to discuss the symptoms with the GP in the first instance.

Chapter Twenty-Nine: Habits of Depressed People

An article on the website Medical News (2019) explores the ways people with depression try to hide it. I felt it would be an interesting exercise to look at those habits and relate them to my own experience.

Firstly, those of us who have struggled with it know the efforts we go to in order to hide it from others, especially when we feel people will not be so understanding. In my own journey, just because I choose to be open about it, does not mean I will not hide how I'm feeling if I think it's appropriate.

1. Talent and Expressive

This essentially suggests that those who are expressive are at higher risk of depression. If we look at the meaning of the word, it is essentially the ability to convey an emotion. Having looked at some biographies of some well-known people who had at least some depressive episodes in their lives, I do believe there may be some merit to this statement. As a writer, I do tend to be more in tune with emotions, both positive and negative. I often felt in my work as a journalist that I was able to understand both sides of an argument.

However, this does not mean just 'creative' or 'artistic' people get depression. Athletes, healthcare professionals, or those who work in the legal profession, are not necessarily 'expressive' in that sense.

2. High Defence Mechanisms

This talks about people building walls around themselves. Having heard a friend tell me I've had walls up, I can believe it. When I am going through a bad patch, I tend to withdraw emotionally. I have had this happen several times, particularly when work has been stressful. I would refuse to talk to my colleagues unless it pertained to work.

Having said that, I am not very good at hiding my emotions. Most people who know me are well aware when I am not happy.

3. Issues with Abandonment

When you have depression, the last thing you want to do is be a burden on someone. With that in mind, it is really difficult to allow people into your life. Depression is you at your worst, and you feel that you cannot reasonably expect someone to have to put up with that.

I have known people with this who have lost friends because those friends cannot deal with it. Having had similar experiences with family members, I tend to push people away rather than let them in because I am afraid that they will decide I am not worth it. I tell myself that if my friends wanted a relationship with me, they would make an effort. It is a two-way street.

There is a famous quote by Marilyn Monroe. "If you cannot handle me at my worst, then you don't deserve me at my best."

4. Weird Eating Habits

I have always had poor nutritional habits. Some of it is out of fear, while the rest of it is habit. When I am feeling low, I turn to junk food – potato chips, chocolate, sweets. It does release certain chemicals like endorphins, but ultimately, it makes me feel worse because I put on weight, or it causes problems with my digestive system. It becomes a vicious circle.

I have known others who have craved unhealthy food at their lowest points. As will be explored in the chapter on nutrition, poor eating habits can lead to depressive moods. However, as mentioned above, consumption of it can lead to the release of 'feel-good' chemicals. However, it should be noted that the effect is temporary.

5. Weird Sleeping Habits

It can be staying up too late or getting up too early. It can mean bouts of insomnia or sleeping in the afternoons – all of which have happened to me.

As the article states, rest is one of the things that someone with depression can have a bit of control over when everything else seems out of control. However, rest does not necessarily mean sleeping. It can mean just closing your eyes and laying down for ten minutes.

6. Over-Thinking Things

This one goes without saying. If I am especially anxious about something, I will go over scenarios in my head, trying to think of the worst that could possibly happen. It makes for many sleepless hours. I have been told not to over-think things, or that I am thinking too negatively, which rankles.

I also tend to think about incidents in the past and continually beat myself up about them. This is, as mentioned in the previous chapter, the inner critic. This is not unusual for most people, but I think people like me tend to make more of them than is really needed.

Sometimes when I am posting something online and someone makes a comment that doesn't sit well, I tend to over-think what they meant and take the more negative view of it instead of shrugging it off as something that came out the wrong way.

7. Self-Reliant

When I have certain problems, like financial difficulties, it is hard for me to accept help, even from family. There is also the other side of it where I think that I am wasting my time asking for help because I usually do not get it. Pride is also a major factor in the refusal to ask for help.

8. Always Ready for the Worst

This fits in with number six above. We think of the worst-case scenario and expect it. When we are told we're being too negative, we get defensive.

9. Habitual Remedies

Keeping to a certain routine is important to someone with depression as it allows for some sense of control even when everything else is out of our control. Whether it is going for a walk at a certain time, or getting up for breakfast at a certain time, it allows us to get into a certain frame of mind. Often, if something bad happens at the start of the day, throwing out our routine, it can feel like a portent for the rest of the day. This can sometimes be a self-fulfilling prophecy in the sense that if we think the day is going to be bad based on that first event, then it will be.

10. Cover-Up Stories

Some days, if I am feeling down, I will either do my best to avoid people or I will just tell them "I'm not feeling well". It is a small thing, but again, it comes down to what we think people can handle. It can give us a sense of control.

11. Heightened Perception of Life and Death

The article states that in a moment of crisis, someone with depression becomes very aware of their mortality. I cannot really say for sure if I have ever felt this, although in my darkest moments, I will admit I do feel as if people would be better off if I were not around.

12. Intense Understanding of Substances

This is something I do know quite a bit about. I worry about the effects of certain substances, and I am not talking about various narcotics. I have studied the effects of various things like coffee, Coca-Cola, vitamins and prescribed medication in-depth. Again, it's a sense of control.

13. Searching for a Purpose

We all wonder what we're put on this Earth for. When you have depression, you constantly ask yourself: 'Why me?'. As if there is some lesson that we are supposed to learn from our experience.

We do want some kind of validation, but this is not uncommon. We just appear to question it more than others.

14. Seek Love and Acceptance

This is related to issues of abandonment. We think we have to present our best side at all times so we will be loved and accepted by our friends and family.

One of the toughest things at times is the feeling that our family cannot accept what is happening with us and it can lead to further feelings of isolation.

15. Subtle Cries for Help

Most of the time we tend to withdraw and not want to be around others, so on the instances where we do want to be around others, it's usually assumed it's because we're in a good place. Unfortunately, that is not always true.

I was going through a bad patch and I was restless and crying. I didn't want to be in my space and sought help from a friend. I didn't even have to say anything she was just there for me when I needed her.

16. Lifestyle Changes

When I have been at my worst, I have tried to think of ways to make changes in my life to help myself get better. This sometimes means I will go out for long walks. This does not necessarily mean it is a bad thing. It is just a strategy people employ to help them manage. It is a little like someone who wants to lose weight decides to throw out all the bad foods in their pantry and get a bit of exercise. They are doing what they need to, to help themselves feel better.

17. Avoidance

When I share living quarters with someone, sometimes it is just easier to avoid them when I am not feeling my best, rather than try to talk to them about what is going on. I do not usually avoid my responsibilities but if I can avoid doing something, I will. On a similar note, I will avoid social things if at all possible when I am not feeling up to it.

18. Compulsive Behaviours

Some people may begin to exhibit compulsive behaviours, but this is something I have not really noticed about myself. These can be anything from taking showers more frequently, washing hands several times a day, or sitting and doing nothing but one activity the entire day.

19. Steering Conversations Away From Themselves

Some people do not like talking about themselves. While this is not a huge problem for me, the truth is, I am not good at talking about anything. Unless someone asks me what is going on, I usually do not volunteer information about myself. Or I will get a 'bee in my bonnet' and talk almost incessantly on one subject. It is another way of avoidance, I think.

20. Avoiding Eye Contact

It is suggested that this is due to a sense of low self-esteem. Looking directly at someone can be disconcerting when you have any type of social anxiety.

21. Reacting Unexpectedly Negatively

Sometimes I will have sudden outbursts. Usually, it is because there has been something bothering me, and I have been stewing on it for a while. I have learnt not to let it stew, although it takes practice, and I do not always get it right.

Most of the time, these outbursts are not because a person with depression is in a bad mood. It just means there is something on their mind, and they have no other way of expressing it.

22. Disappearing for Long Periods

There are times when I need to 'get out of my headspace'. A change of scenery can help with that.

There was one incident where I decided to take a drive out to the beach. It was at least a half-hour drive, and it helped to clear my head a little.

If someone in your family does this on a fairly frequent basis, it is probably a sign that they are not coping.

Chapter Thirty: Myths about depression

1.   Depression is a part of the 'human condition'.

The human condition is described as characteristics, key events and situations which make up the essentials of human existence.

The one thing I find a little disturbing about this statement is that depression is 'normal'. To feel depressed about something that has happened and move on is 'normal', but to my mind, depression is not. These are two totally separate conditions.

While the feeling of depression itself is essentially a human condition, in that every human being with the capability of feeling emotions is bound to feel depressed at one time or another, the statement grossly simplifies the fact that the illness, as described by the medical community, comes from a complex series of human behaviours, emotions and, in some cases, physiological and mental conditions.

Some have suggested that the feeling of depression is actually a 'choice', not an illness. Having been through bouts of depression and suicidal ideations many times in my life, I have to question this idea.

First, let's address the latter. Some articles suggest that describing it as an 'illness' implies that those with depression need to go on medication. As I will explore in later chapters, medication is not always the best option for some, while others will feel differently. There is no right or wrong when it comes to medication. I choose not to use anti-depressants and would rather just follow a plan of nutrition and exercise. As I will explore in more detail later, who is to say that nutrition is not a form of medication in itself? As Hippocrates supposedly said: 'Let food be thy medicine and let medicine be thy food'.

However, I should point out that this is my personal choice. Others may decide to use medication along with following a nutrition and exercise plan, and there is nothing at all wrong with that.

I certainly did not choose to have depression. Some articles I have read suggest that we do have the option to change the way we feel or respond to either the depression or the situations which cause that depression and while that is true, it is not always that simple.

As an example, I have had experiences of negative feelings and thoughts, not just from myself, but from others. Yes, I can choose how I respond to those negative comments, but it can be difficult when the messages are constant.

To use an analogy, imagine being bombarded with a television advertisement that is so irritating that you are either turning the sound off or changing the channel. Only, in some cases, to find that the same advertisement is on another channel. As a child, I would see such advertisements that were so   irritating I would mock them at every opportunity. To this day, I can still remember them almost by heart.

I have described my depression as having an angel self on one shoulder and a devil self on the other, rather like those Disney cartoons where Donald Duck has the same characters. Both are telling him different things, like: 'be good, Donald', or 'go ahead and do that bad thing, you know you want to'. In my case, the angel is telling me I am a good person, that I am smart, caring, compassionate, etc., etc. Whereas, the devil is telling me I am not good enough, that I am ugly, I deserve every bad thing that is happening to me, and so on.

So, these two characters are constantly fighting with each

other, each one getting progressively louder and louder until I essentially can't hear myself think. That, coupled with negative messages from my father, bullies undermining my self-esteem, and strangers in the street yelling out rude comments which also undermine my self-esteem, it is little wonder I cannot 'see the forest for the trees'.

Perhaps I did have a choice in how I responded to these people, but again, it is difficult to shrug off such things when the messages are constant.

In my view, that is not a natural part of being human. To reiterate the point, the actual illness is far more complex than that.

2.   Depression is just Sadness

Most people tend to believe that depression is just 'being sad'. There is a quote from Henry Wadsworth Longfellow which says that 'everyone has secret sorrows ... oftentimes we call a man cold when he is merely sad'. Longfellow is also quoted as saying: 'Into each life, some rain must fall' (Longfellow, 1842).

This does not even begin to compare to what depression actually is. While there is an element of sadness, it is not prevalent in all cases.

Dictionary.com defines sadness as: 'affected by unhappiness or grief', or 'causing sorrow', but depression is much more than sorrow, as described in the point above.

Most feelings of sadness are only temporary, whereas depression is chronic and long-lasting.

3.   Depression is 'trendy'

To say something is trendy implies something is 'cool' or 'in'. To people with depression, it is definitely not cool, and if they had a choice, they certainly would not choose to have it.

There is a line from the tv show *Buffy the Vampire Slayer* which illustrates the point about 'trends' in such illnesses. One of the main characters, Cordelia, is talking about her mother, who has a chronic illness which prevents her from even getting out of bed. Cordelia complains that the illness is not the latest 'trendy' illness and that it is not cool (Whedon, 1997).

The fact that the above illnesses have been dismissed by some as 'not real' is something they have in common with depression.

There are some who feel that because there is more awareness around depression, it means it has become 'trendy'. Like, various illnesses such as chronic fatigue, the reason they are mentioned more is because more is known about them.

Mental health is a topic that generally used to be ignored, or people tried to pretend it didn't exist. That comes down to a perception that dates back to when anyone with any kind of mental health issue was committed to an asylum.

Nowadays, it is more socially acceptable to be open about it, although there is still much work to be done before it will be fully accepted as a real illness.

4.   Talking about it makes it worse

While this is more generally about suicide, there are some people who suggest that being more open about depression and anxiety makes the problem worse. Anecdotal evidence from sufferers is that the opposite is true. Some would say people shouldn't mention it to all and sundry, and while this may be true, it is generally a good idea to at least be open about it.

There has always been a certain stigma around depression but talking about it opens up a discussion and promotes more understanding.

I do not usually mention my own depression to strangers unless it comes up as a topic of discussion, but I do not close myself off to it either. I may mention it in passing, not with the expectation that those around me will feel sorry for me, but so they will understand why I act the way I do. For instance, I can go to a party and sit there without saying anything, yet I will not appear to be enjoying myself. This is just who I am and no reflection on the party or the guests. However, I will not come out and say: "I have depression" in such a setting.

Talking about what we go through not only helps us understand ourselves, but helps others to understand us as well, rather than us being labelled as weird, or 'anti-social'.

I have also experienced the other side of it where it feels that people do not want to hear about my 'problems'. That usually makes me withdraw and internalise my feelings until it comes to a point where I will feel so low, I will want to do something drastic (i.e. suicidal ideations) or I will 'blow' (i.e. lose my temper).

5.   Depression/mental illness means I'm crazy

Some people believe that anyone with depression, major or minor, is crazy. There is historical evidence that around 50 years ago, those with mental illnesses were locked up in psychiatric institutions. Even now, some patients with major depressive episodes seeking help from hospitals find themselves in rather dreary conditions, which often make them feel worse. This has mostly been due to the lack of funding for mental health services leading to a lower level of care, although the current government is trying to remedy that.

There have been several shootings in recent years, particularly in the United States, and it is often mentioned that the shooter had 'mental health issues'. This can lead to more stigma about mental illness as a whole. However, it should be noted that hundreds of thousands of people are diagnosed with mental illness every year, and the majority do not go out and commit violent crimes.

Psych Central founder and editor-in-chief Dr John M. Grohol states in his blog that, while depression is a serious mental disorder, most mental disorders are just as serious (Grohol, 2018).

6.   Only losers or old people get depression

Depression does not discriminate. Statistics show that it can affect anyone, young or old. Who they are, regardless of their perceived level of success, their age, their social status or their financial position, is completely irrelevant. As will be noted later, even those who are at the height of personal success can get depression.

Similarly, while more women seem to be diagnosed with depression, this does not necessarily mean more women than men have it. Diagnosis depends on various factors. Dr Grohol says that there is a belief that men should not show any weakness, so seeking help or a diagnosis may not be an option. The fact that some men are taught not to seek such help can skew statistics.

Depression is also not a normal part of ageing. The government enquiry into mental health found that children and young people were experiencing mental health problems to a high degree (He Ara Oranga, NZ Government, 2018). Statistics taken from the health survey 2017 estimated around 79,000 between the ages of 15 and 24 had been diagnosed with depression (Ministry of Health 2016-17). While the numbers were higher in other age brackets it shows that it is not just older people who have depression.

7.   The patient will have to take medication for life

Most people believe that once they have been prescribed anti-depressants, they will have to take them for the rest of their life. This is not necessarily the case. It may depend on the severity of the depressive episodes. Treatment periods vary depending on how well the patient learns different coping strategies.

GP David Hill from the Health Hub Project in Palmerston North believes in taking a holistic approach and says medication is "sometimes useful, but not always".

Anti-depressants are a common treatment, but it is often a question of which will work better. There are a variety of these medications, but it does depend on the patient. My belief is that it is a matter of personal choice.

8.   'Suck it up, buttercup'

Depression is not something we can just 'get over'. It cannot be repeated enough. There is no cure for it. Those who say they can beat depression may feel they have, but there may be times when symptoms can return.

Like other debilitating illnesses, the symptoms are managed with various strategies. Unfortunately, for most of us, 'getting over it' is not simply a matter of just getting out of bed and refusing to acknowledge the negative feelings.

There have been a few memes through social media on this topic, illustrating exactly this point. Would you tell someone in a wheelchair to just 'get over it'? Like the person in the wheelchair, patients with depression have their good days and bad days, but it still does not mean they can pretend the condition doesn't exist or that they can suddenly decide not to have it.

9.   Depression is just negative thinking

I have been told this many times, and my answer is always the same. It is not that simple. Some might suggest that negative thinking causes depression, but it is not always the case for most people. Sometimes it is a case of which came first, the chicken or the egg? Or: the negative thinking or the depression? The question needs to be asked: can we really blame a negative outlook for depression?

In my own experience, I have been told I am 'too negative', but I cannot with all certainty point to that as the crux of the problem.

An article in *Psychology Today* (Marano, 2016) explores this further.

10.   You got depression from your parent(s)

While there are cases in which there is a proven family history of mental illness, a causal relationship cannot be firmly established. It may be that children have a genetic predisposition to it; however, the chances of them actually getting it are very small and dependent on other factors before genetics should even be considered.

11.   You can 'pull yourself out of depression'

Suggesting we can pull ourselves out of depression is akin to implying that we choose to have depression. If that was the case, this is the last thing anyone would want.

It is far more complicated than that and researchers in Behavioural Science also state that there are complex relationships at work between the brain and how it is affected by its environment, both internally and externally (Abrams, 2018).

12.   You can't have depression if you're successful

This is similar to point six above. Someone like former All Black Sir John Kirwan would disagree. Not to mention many other well-known artists, musicians, actors, doctors, scientists, politicians and the like. Depression can happen to anyone, at any time.

On a similar note, when an apparently successful or even famous person reveals they struggle with depression, they are told they should be 'grateful' for what they have. Depression is not about being ungrateful. For some, it may be a matter of them feeling guilty for the life they do have. Depression compounds that guilt.

I once wrote something in a work of fiction that is relevant here. No one 'deserves' the life they are born into, whether it is someone who is born into abject poverty or the child of the richest man on Earth. The point is what they do with the life they are given.

Chapter Thirty-One: What Causes Depression?

Why do some people get depression and others don't? Why can some people seem to shrug off various negative or painful incidents in their life and not feel like their entire world has come crashing down? What makes one person's experience with depression different from another's?

There are many theories of what causes depression and just as many debates. Some psychologists prefer the 'chemical imbalance' argument while others suggest environmental factors are to blame. More might argue that we are too quick to blame depression when it might be something else entirely.

It is true that there is a risk depression may be mistakenly diagnosed as the cause of a person's illness when it could be something else. Is it being 'over-diagnosed'? It is difficult to say. I must emphasise that diagnosis is subjective, in that a doctor must rely on both the patient's perception of their state of health and on various guidelines they are given. However, this can be true of other illnesses that cannot be simply diagnosed by pathological means. It also requires total honesty from the patient; for instance, if they are a drug user, this may affect their emotional state.

There is a plethora of research now available into what causes depression, but it would be foolish to lay the blame purely at the feet of one thing. Through an analysis of my own illness, I can see that it is not just things like low self-esteem, or my response to stress.

In this chapter, I will explore some of the causes and in some cases, use my own experiences to illustrate them.

The first part deals with some research into clinical studies. This is important, as it explores some of the theories involving brain and behaviour. These are only some of the theories around that experts turn to when trying to explain what causes depression. However, as I try to illustrate in the second part, there are other factors.

The important thing to remember is that everyone's situation is different and that the following theories may not apply in all cases. Another thing to consider is context. Those psychologists who follow the Freudian school of thought will understand that it is the events in a person's life, or their environment that should be considered as factors in depression; while others will still follow the theory that there is a physiological or biological culprit at work. However, to the best of my knowledge, there is no known accurate method of diagnosis which would provide a definitive answer.

Psychiatrists use what some would call a 'bible' of mental health: The Diagnostic and Statistical Manual of Mental Disorders (DSM5) (2013). Released by the American Psychiatric Association, it provides guidelines and describes symptoms and other criteria for diagnosing mental illnesses. Its guidelines for depression state that symptoms must be present for at least two weeks.

As some of these theories are fairly technical, I thought it would be necessary to provide some definitions.

Hippocampus

The word itself comes from Greek. Hippo means horse, and kampo means monster. It is found in the bottom middle section of the brain known as the temporal lobe.

The hippocampus' main functions involve human learning

and memory (Dresden, 2019). It is also vulnerable to damage from various things such as stress.

Hypothalamus

A small region of the brain located at the base, near the pituitary gland. Its functions include releasing hormones, regulating body temperature, appetite control, and emotional responses (Saladi-Schulman, 2018).

Lateral Habenula

A part of the brain which regulates motivational states (Nuno-Perez et al, 2018). Simply put, it sends signals to the body telling it how to react to certain situations.

Cortisol

A hormone which controls blood sugar levels, acts as an anti-inflammatory and influences blood pressure (Society for Endocrinology 2019).

Neuro-transmitters

Chemicals which act as the brain's messengers, carrying signals from one neuron to the other via the body's nervous system. Two neurotransmitters which may be familiar are serotonin and dopamine.

1. **Brain research**

We now have various technologies available which can help doctors get a closer look at the brain to try to figure out what is happening in someone who has depression, compared to someone who hasn't. Such things as positron emission tomography (PET), single-photon emission computed tomography (SPECT); and functional magnetic resonance imaging (fMRI) has been used in these instances.

I queried this with theoretical neuroscientist Professor Mark Humphries. "These kinds of studies that use MRI to compare the volumes of brain structures between patients and controls are always difficult to interpret. They lack any theoretical motivation, and so are largely just reporting differences they have noticed. But by testing a large number of differences, and only reporting those that reach 'significance', such studies are bound to find some difference." (Humphries, email, 2019)

Some researchers have found that the hippocampus is smaller in depressed people. One such study investigated women with a history of depression and discovered that the hippocampus was smaller in those women compared with others who did not have depression (Harvard Health Publishing, 2009).

Other studies have been done with those prescribed with PTSD (Post-traumatic Stress Disorder), with similar findings.

The findings above are relevant to a TED talk mentioned in the chapter on fitness in the next section. However, these findings should be taken with the proverbial grain of salt. Explore it further and look into some other research around the size of the hippocampus and see if that research has come up with links to different illnesses or disease.

Other researchers suggest depression is the result of 'maladaptive changes in specific brain circuits' (Yan Yang, et al, 2019). Simply put, those brain circuits aren't responding appropriately in given situations.

In an article on the search for the culprit in depression, Professor Humphries states that the brain has 86 billion neurons (2018, used with permission). Some of those neurons are part of the problem. The question is which. Professor Humphries points to the lateral habenula.

This particular region is responsible for the body's reactions to stimulus, or lack thereof. Where we might normally react to something pleasant or unexpected, the lateral habenula basically tells the body that everything is normal. In depression, one of the chief characteristics is the inability to feel pleasure.

How it works is the body contains neurotransmitters such as dopamine and serotonin. These are, in simple terms, the body's messengers, carrying signals via the nervous system to neurons, or from the neurons to the muscles.

The above neurotransmitters are loosely known as 'happy pills' for the brain and are most often linked with depression.

Dopamine becomes activated when something good happens (Newton, 2019). It's also considered a reward chemical.

Dopamine is known to help with motivation, purpose and drive. It is released when we are about to achieve something, and our needs are about to be met as well as once they are met. It is commonly known for affecting our emotions and our sensations of pleasure and pain. There are various clinical trials which study dopamine and its effects.

Experts state serotonin is a natural mood stabiliser, helping to reduce anxiety and depression as well as improving sleep, digestion and sexual function.

It is generally thought that depression can be caused by low levels of serotonin, for one. Such low levels are caused by a deficiency of an amino acid called tryptophan, which can be found in the diet (Scaccia, 2017).

In a normal brain, "When dopamine neurons burst with activity, that's a signal we just got something better than expected," Professor Humphries explains in his article. "And when the lateral habenula releases a burst of activity, it stops the dopamine and serotonin neurons from bursting. Stops them from telling the brain: 'Hey, that was unexpected'."

Which is all good in a normal brain. So, what happens when someone is depressed?

Scientists conducted experiments using depressed rats and mice, but found the neurons were bursting too much, sending the wrong signals, so the brain was not reacting as it should.

Essentially, what the lateral habenula does in someone with depression is rob the brain of its access to both neurotransmitters.

In looking further for a reason why this happens, Professor Humphries points to the culprit, otherwise known as the Glia. Glia, or glial cells provide support for neurons. When they go wrong, in the case of depression, they are depleting the body's reserves of potassium, "making its neuron neighbour depressed, so depressed it bursts when it should not; and this bursting is, it seems, a cause of what we call depression."

Trials have been performed using a medication known as Ketamine. Originally, this was used an anaesthetic, but has been trialled as a treatment for depression since the early 2000s. An article in The Guardian stated that a drug called Esketamine has now been approved by the US Food and Drug Administration (Glenza, 2019).

The problem is that Ketamine may not work for everyone. Which may indicate that these faulty neurons are not the only culprit.

2. Genetics

Scientists have identified genes which may help in identifying those who may have a predisposition toward depression (Harvard, 2009).

Every part of the body is controlled by genes, which turn on and off as needed. But sometimes those genes get things wrong, which creates havoc on moods.

A goal of gene research is not just to find out how to treat depression, but also to understand why some people are more vulnerable to depression. It is well-known that mental health issues tend to run in families. In my own case, as I mentioned earlier, while it was never actually diagnosed, I have always had a suspicion my father had depression.

Research on bipolar disorder (otherwise known as manic depression) has helped in identifying the genetics involved.

In studies on twins, it was found that in identical twins, if one twin had bipolar, the other twin had a very high likelihood of also developing it. In fraternal twins, the chances were much lower; the difference being that identical twins share a genetic blueprint (Harvard, 2009).

However, genetics is only one of many key players. As mentioned earlier, a causal relationship between genetics and depression cannot be firmly established in some cases, as there are many other variables that need to be considered.

3.   Stress

Stress also plays a key role in the way the brain behaves, affecting such areas as the hippocampus.

Studies have been done with patients with PTSD. While this has been around for a few decades, originally it was more likely thought to be 'shell shock' or combat fatigue, as the symptoms are similar.

PTSD is usually considered to be something only those who have been in combat experienced, which is understandable. Some of the earlier research has been around those who fought in Vietnam. However, this kind of stress disorder can also occur for someone who has been involved in an accident, a house fire, or even experienced physical or sexual abuse. Symptoms are generally anxiety, as well as depression in some cases.

Having experienced major stress in my life, I can attest to this causal relationship. One of the things that people noticed with my own issues was that when I was at my lowest point, I had difficulty coping with the stress I was under. I did learn some strategies to manage it, however.

It is not always easy. I still get stressed out, especially over financial issues, which makes it difficult for my immediate family. It may sound to others like I am angry at my family for the situation I find myself in, but it is more that I am angry at myself for not being able to find my own solution to it without having to ask for help.

We are all aware of some of the problems stress can cause. For instance, it raises cortisol levels in the blood and can lead to weight gain. Some chronic conditions are treated with steroids and in some patients, causes weight gain or at the very least, puffiness.

The Society of Endocrinology has an educational resource online which explains the function of cortisol. This is a hormone which has a number of functions including controlling blood sugar levels, acting as an anti-inflammatory and influencing blood pressure, to name a few.

Extra cortisol is released which helps the body to respond to stressful situations (Society for Endocrinology, 2019).

If there is too much cortisol over a long period of time, it can lead to something called Cushing's Syndrome, which includes symptoms such as high blood pressure and mood swings.

This is one way to illustrate the chemical reactions that occur within the body when dealing with stress.

We all experience stressful situations at some point in our lives, whether it is losing a job, illness, the death of a loved one. Yet some people are able to manage it and move on, while others are unable to cope. It may stem from the length of time a person is under stress. For instance, in my case, being in and out of work, dealing with parental abuse, or being constantly bullied over long periods can add up to major stress.

Recent studies have also found that bullying in the work place can also lead to lower productivity, brought on by low self-esteem, or self-doubt.

When I have been able to get a job and feel a little more financially stable, my depression, while not quite going away, becomes more manageable.

Again, genetics does have a role to play in stress, as some people are naturally wired to be more sensitive to such things. Being a sensitive person myself, I know that the stressful situations I have faced have affected my performance at work, and impacts on my ability to interact positively with my family and friends.

You may have heard of the 'fight or flight' response. This was a theory first postulated by American physiologist Walter Bradford Cannon (Wikipedia, biography). The fight or flight response is the body's natural reaction to perceived threats.

Most people would know that this more than likely dates back to when man had to hunt for food, so they would have to be ready to protect themselves from predators. Nowadays, of course, we live different lives, so the threats are completely different, yet our bodies react in much the same way. It is when it overreacts that it becomes a problem.

Normally once the threat has gone, we should be able to turn off those defences. However, in some cases, that does not happen, leading to physiological problems such as high blood pressure, immune suppression and depression, to name a few (Harvard, 2009).

Researchers are now looking into why these 'over-reactions' occur. The best illustration of this is in those who experience hayfever, or allergic rhinitis. When pollen enters the nasal passages, the body creates histamine against the invader. In a hayfever sufferer, the immune system overreacts, causing the person to sneeze.

The hypothalamus also plays a part in the stress response. When a threat, whether physical or emotional, looms, it secretes a hormone which rouses the body, prompting the release of cortisol. It's a little more complicated than that, involving various pathways within the body.

The particular hormone of interest is called a corticotropin-releasing hormone, or CRH. Scientists believe this plays a major role in co-ordinating thoughts and behaviours, as well as emotional reactions. Studies have found that people with depression have increased levels of this hormone (Harvard, 2009).

4. Medical conditions

Some medical conditions have also been known to lead to mood disorders. There are theories that problems with the thyroid are one of them. One person I spoke to did experience such an issue when part of her thyroid was removed, leading to a diagnosis of bipolar disorder.

I once consulted a nutritionist who told me after looking at blood tests that I had an under-active thyroid, otherwise known as hypo-thyroidism. Some research suggests that this may be a cause of depression in some people. However, in my case, it would be difficult to establish a causal relationship given that my depression was diagnosed long before I was told about my thyroid.

Doctors also know that some chronic health conditions also cause depression in some people. In an online course run through King's College in London, one of the examples they used was someone undergoing dialysis. This led to a disconnection of sorts as the man had to be at the hospital for hours each time, which took time away from his employment, his friends and family. Adding to the low moods was a broken marriage and not being able to see his child.

This was probably a dramatization but much of the information used in the course would have come from real-life examples. While not every person with a chronic illness will have the same problems, it is a good way to illustrate what some patients go through.

There are other causes of depression which I have learnt through my own analysis.

5. Guilt

One of the major issues with my own depression was that I always felt guilty for the problems in my family.

I considered myself a jinx. It was not just the issues with my birth, of which there were many, but it was the hurtful way I was treated that led me to make such conclusions.

There are a few examples I can name. One major incident comes to mind, of when my brother started high school. He was given a brand-new bicycle when he was old enough. I learnt many years later that my mother had given my father money to buy a new cycle for me as well when I had outgrown my old one. Instead, he bought an old one and painted it up to look new. It was far from modern. This was the mid-1980s when it was becoming more common to have bicycles with gears.

My father had taken the simple gear mechanism from an old Raleigh 20, which had a two-speed hub where you could shift gears via the pedals and installed it on the refurbished bicycle. Yet my brother's new bicycle had the more modern cable gears - in those days only about three gears but still far better in my view. I can only imagine what he used the money for.

We always had money problems. My brother and I were born in the same month, but two years and 11 days apart. When I was twelve, my mother got a job where she was paid on a fortnightly basis. Unfortunately, my birthday always fell in a 'non-pay' week. While my brother got his birthday presents on the day, there were many occasions I had to wait until the next pay week. This probably makes me sound a bit spoiled, but when you are a child, especially a lonely child like myself, birthdays have a huge significance. Celebrating your 'special day' a day or two later just does not have the same meaning. It also felt like my brother was more important than I was, even though the timing of his birth was hardly his fault.

The interesting thing was, when my parents briefly separated, and my mother was on a benefit, she managed to save some money. There were never any savings with my father around since it was all spent on gambling.

I often felt my family would have been better off if I had not been born. My father, I am sure, knew of this, but never did anything to disabuse me of that notion.

Other people may feel guilt for other reasons: some may be linked to grief. For instance, a family member may have died through what may seem like something that was preventable. When something like this happens, it is natural for a person to wish they could reverse time and bring that person back. It is when those natural feelings turn to long-term depression that it becomes a problem.

6.   Environment

We all know of the nature-versus-nurture debate, but it is true that we are a product of our environment. This, coupled with a lack of encouragement from a major influence in one's life, is also a factor in depression.

Abuse is another. While some would argue physical abuse is worse, I would place emotional abuse on a par with it. The problem with emotional abuse is that it can be subtle, so that the person being abused may not even be aware that it is happening until someone else points it out to them. My father's possessiveness, apparent chauvinistic attitude and his negativity were constants in my life, and it is only now that he has passed that I can actually see his treatment for what it was.

7.   Self-esteem

As I have mentioned before, I have always had a low sense of self-esteem. This is also a major factor in depression in a lot of people.

I have often been asked why I consider myself unattractive. Part of it is due to my lack of confidence. Another part is my inability to fit in with my perception of what the world expects.

I have memories of my maternal grandmother asking me from the age of 17 when I was getting a boyfriend, when I was getting married, etcetera.

If I take a step back, I can sort of understand her attitude. She was born in the early 1920s when feminism wasn't really heard of as a movement back then. Much of the advertising from that era was focused on women looking beautiful for their husbands, cooking, cleaning, raising children. Despite the fact that many of the men went off to fight in the Second World War by the time she was of 'child-bearing age', it was still considered normal for a woman to stay at home and raise the family rather than go out to work. Yes, women did work, either because their husbands had joined the fighting, they were separated, or they were widows. Single women tended to work until they got married.

This is by no means an accurate picture of how life really was back in the forties, but in general, this was how I believe most women were taught to think.

I grew up at the beginning of the feminist movement. I still remember in the eighties, when I was a teenager, the slogan: 'Girls can do anything'. My generation was at the forefront of that movement and at the very beginnings of change when it was seen to be possible that girls really could do anything.

We often see it in the media. During my teenage years, we saw the rise of the 'supermodel'. Christie Brinkley, Claudia Schiffer, Naomi Campbell, Cindy Crawford, Linda Evangelista and New Zealand's own Rachel Hunter were the women on whose standards we were all judged. Let's face it. Looking like them, without the help of make-up artists and photographers to air brush out any flaws, would be downright impossible.

Even I aspired to be like those women. I still look at make-up tutorials on YouTube and wish I had the skills the girls in the tutorials have to hide all my flaws (of which I consider I have many).

The point must be made that beauty is a social construction. By that, I mean that we believe society decides what is acceptable. They are fundamental beliefs and values within a certain framework. For example, western society's beliefs on what beauty is. Have you ever looked at some videos on YouTube showing images of every culture's idea of what a beautiful woman looks like? This is what I mean by a social construct. Ask yourself: who decides this? Did they go out and survey random people on the street for their opinion?

These constructs change with every new generation. For instance, actress Marilyn Monroe. In her time, she was considered a beautiful, curvaceous woman, but by today's standards she would be considered 'plus-sized'. Just a few years after her death, a woman nicknamed Twiggy (Lesley Lawson) was considered the standard. Twiggy was known for a very thin build and androgynous looks.

Twenty years later, and models were judged on their stick-thin or almost anorexic builds. Basically, the thinner, the better. However, not too many years after that, many model agencies, magazines and the media received some nasty backlash over the fact that this image was causing many young girls to starve themselves, leading to anorexia or bulimia.

Despite that backlash, today, the media still tends to err on the side of the 'ideal image'. Many magazines have been criticised for 'photoshopping' images of actors or models and various social media platforms have turned these 'fails' into memes.

It is true that I can modify my response to these things and view them with a healthy dose of cynicism. Yet I still judge myself harshly.

What we need to be aware of is that someone out there felt they had the authority and the know-how to decide the standard by which we judge people. The problem with self-esteem occurs when we follow that person's judgement as if it is a hard-and-fast rule, and nothing else can measure up.

8. Self-worth or Success

In many ways, the world still sees the ideal as the 'nuclear family' of two parents, two children. Usually, that means a heterosexual couple with children. When a person has none of these things, they are judged for their value to society, as if having children is the 'be all and end all'.

I measure my own success not only on whether or not I am in a relationship, but I also measure it by my material wealth. I find it difficult to give myself credit for what I have achieved, like my education and having written and published several novels. It is called tunnel vision. When you have depression, your worldview is based on your perception of what people are thinking.

For example, when you meet someone new, what is usually one of the first things they ask you? "What do you do for a living?" As if having an important job (or any job) is what makes you 'worthy' of their attention. They may respond positively or negatively, but again, that may be subjective, based on your perception of their response.

It all comes down to a feeling of being 'not good enough'. We measure ourselves against a yardstick that is actually just an illusion, or in many ways, as above, a social construct. We allow others to bring us down and undermine our self-confidence.

9. Toxic Relationships

This is why people like my dad, and all the bullies in my life, still have a certain power over me. While a big part of me knows they are just projections of their own problems, in that they feel the need to drag others down to their level, another part tries to tell me that 'I deserve it'.

When we are surrounded by people who are basically just bullies, whether they put you down, or talk over you as if they believe they are smarter than you, it can become toxic.

We cannot rule out social media, either. There are stories of young teenagers being bullied via Facebook and Twitter, which can lead to depression, or worse. Unfortunately, until the owners of such sites step up and take some of the responsibility, there is no easy answer to this problem.

This kind of toxicity is one that can be managed if we have the tools to do so.

Another example of a toxic relationship is a spousal one. We can only guess why someone chooses to stay in a relationship where the partner is constantly undermining their 'significant other's' sense of self-worth, self-esteem or confidence or subjecting them to either physical or emotional abuse.

I often see people in various social media groups talking about how their partner is constantly putting them down and making them feel worthless. It is not easy leaving such a relationship. There are many reasons for it. If there are children in the relationship, they may feel the children will be negatively impacted by the separation. They may not have enough money to manage on their own. They may not want others to think they have failed. They may feel that not being part of a 'couple' may invalidate themselves as a person.

Some people might get into relationships to feel less lonely. We fear losing that sense of connection – disconnection is something that will be discussed in a later point. However, if the relationship is a toxic one, there is no connection, and it is often a case of exchanging one bad situation for another.

10. Financial Stress

Financial stress can come from different sources. For myself, being in and out of work, forced to get the jobseeker benefit and barely able to pay my bills on the low income, let alone buy groceries without help, is not only demoralising but deeply depressing. I doubt that I am the only one feeling this way.

It feels to many struggling to make ends meet that the gap between the rich and the poor is getting wider. However, low wages are not the only cause of financial stress.

Back in the 1920s, society seemed to be doing fairly well. It was an era of apparent prosperity, yet there was a huge problem. People were racking up huge debt on credit in order to look better than their neighbours. This idea of the pursuit of material wealth, or 'keeping up with the Joneses' was depicted in a comic strip in the United Kingdom before World War I.

However, this began to create major sociological problems and culminated in the Great Depression and the Wall Street Crash in 1929.

The gist of what happened on that dark day in New York in October 1929 was that stocks began dropping in value at alarming rates, causing many investors to lose great fortunes. There were many reasons why it happened: some due to industrialisation and problems in the agricultural sector but the main reason was massive debt.

Several investors were said to have committed suicide, having lost not only all their money but their reputations.

What does this have to do with the current prevalence of depression? The simple fact that the Great Depression plunged the world into poverty, leaving many people destitute. Yet for all the harsh lessons in the years of struggle, society today really has not learnt a thing. We are still, as a whole, just as materialistic as ever.

As in the part on self-worth, we perceive that we are judged for what we have (or don't have). The less we have in terms of material wealth, the more we are 'looked down on'. I still remember feeling judged as a child and found wanting because my parents did not own the home they lived in. Never mind the fact that many of my classmates would not have been aware that their parents would probably have gone into considerable debt.

Most people pursue jobs that are less to do with their passion and more to do with how much money they can make. They work long hours or pick up other jobs just so they can afford huge mortgages. They 'work to live' rather than 'live to work'. Again, in the pursuit of materialism. When we value money over morality, selfishness over kindness, it can lead to sociological and psychological problems.

As most of us will have seen from the problems in our major metropolitan areas, especially in New Zealand, house prices have risen so much that first-home buyers have found them out of reach. It is little wonder that rates of depression are higher in these areas considering how many families are struggling even to find decent accommodation. The basic human rights of food, clothing and shelter are becoming out of reach.

11. Disconnection

Johann Hari, in his book, *Lost Connections*, talks about being 'disengaged'. He uses the example of those in what some may consider to be 'dead-end' jobs, in which people are doing the same thing, day in and day out.

He notes that for some people with depression, it is a feeling that nothing you do matters. Or to put it another way, that what you are doing is not real. If you have ever seen the movie *The Matrix*, it depicts a world that is created by a machine and that human beings are plugged in, living imaginary lives. This sense of derealisation sounds very similar to the situation in the movie and is another form of disconnection.

My father was what some would call a 'blue-collar' worker. His job title was as a 'storeman' and his duties rarely varied. In the last job he held, he would be required to check stocks of produce and ensure it was in saleable condition, then would have to deliver the produce to various stores. He worked in a dingy warehouse, or he would be out in a van delivering groceries to some of the customers of each store the company was affiliated with. Most of those deliveries were to elderly ladies who were unable to take their own groceries home, which was probably the better part of the role for him. The rest of the time was mostly mundane work, and I can remember he would come home fairly often with debilitating migraines. He left this job in 1981, and there was no such thing as ergonomics. The work he was doing caused some physiological problems.

After he left work, and my mother began working instead, he became what he laughingly called a 'home executive'. Yet, spending time doing housework, looking after us as children, shopping and cooking meals was hardly a life-affirming role. Given what I now believe to be a rather chauvinistic view of how it is the man who goes out to work, it probably was a huge let-down for him.

He had few friends and became severely disconnected from the rest of the world. His only connection would be through his gambling but even then there was no real socialisation.

In my own experience, I have always had trouble with socialisation. While I was working for a newspaper, I was happy. I liked what I was doing, going out and talking to people for news stories. As shy as I was socially, professionally, it was another matter.

When I began working for another company, I was not allowed to take part in company social activities (other than the annual Christmas party). Anything to do with the larger company affected my position just as much as anyone else. Yet I was not permitted to attend any company-wide meetings either. Once work became extremely busy, I would come in earlier than I was officially supposed to start. There were times in my job when most of the work was done, and I would have nothing to do except wait for communication from customers.

As a journalist, I felt I was making a difference in a small way. I proved this by winning an award for my writing. In my other roles, I was just another cog in the wheel. I was living on my own and had no friends visiting, which no doubt added to my feelings of disconnection.

What was often soul-destroying for me was that the job I was doing once I began working in customer service, didn't stimulate my brain. In essence, it was an insult to my intelligence. I was also not being paid fairly for the amount of work I was doing.

After more than two years of doing the same thing, day in and day out, I felt under-appreciated and certainly abused. I was rarely thanked for my efforts and in most cases, it was a token gesture. For instance, once I reached an anniversary, I was given a card by the CEO and a bottle of wine. Most people would have taken the gesture for how it was meant, but to me, it was offensive. I do not drink. In fact, I hate wine, to the point it makes me nauseous. It felt like no one had actually taken the time to ask about that, so the gesture, as well-meant as I'm sure it was, was pointless. It made me feel that it was just a token and certainly not an effort to show that top management actually cared about their staff.

I was on the same wage in that role when I left as when I started, after more than two years. Given the huge amount of responsibility, that was extremely demoralising and after I had learnt that the temporary employees I was meant to be supervising were paid higher than myself, it added to my feelings of dissatisfaction, compounding my stress and depression.

Now, while I am not working, I do have a sense of connection, as I am involved in a service organisation. The work I do there is recognised in a positive way. Thanks to getting involved in a fandom, it gave me another sense of connection. I also have online friends I talk to on a regular basis and, through my writing I feel I am doing something worthwhile. Therein lies the difference.

12. Diet

Some neuroscientists have studied diet in depth and believe there is a correlation between what people eat and their depression. As mentioned earlier, low levels of potassium can be part of that. Certainly, a lack of the right kind of nutrients can cause changes in mood.

However, it should only be considered a factor as there may be deeper issues involved.

Let's not forget the trend of 'fat shaming' on social media (although I have heard of underweight people also being criticised). I have seen extremely negative comments on various sites relating to a person's weight. Even online communities, where members rant about the rudeness of people, they make disparaging remarks about a person's appearance. While the person being talked about has behaved badly, the member still has no idea why that person is the way they are.

In my experience, my weight gain came about for several reasons, least of which was bad nutrition. I have yet to understand why but I believe that in many ways it was my attempt to keep up the walls my father had caused me to build, afraid that I would get hurt if I let them down.

These are some of the major causes of depression. While there is no easy answer to solve the problems, there are ways to manage the symptoms of depression.

Chapter Thirty-Two: Statistics

While crunching numbers can be boring, statistics can give us a general picture of how prevalent depression is in terms of population.

I did a quick analysis of population statistics in New Zealand and compared it to estimates from the Ministry of Health.

At the time of writing, the statistics from the 2018 Census were unavailable, so I compared numbers from the 2013 Census with the 2013 estimates.

In 2013, New Zealand had a population of around 4.2 million. The table below is from the 2013 Census. Bear in mind that some people identified as more than one ethnicity.

Table 1: **POPULATION BY ETHNICITY – PERCENTAGE**

ETHNICITY	PERCENTAGE
NZ European	67%
Maori	13 %
Pacific	7%
Asian	10.5%
Middle Eastern/Latin American	1%
Other	1.5%

The depression statistics were slightly different. The estimates grouped together NZ European and other ethnicities, and Middle Eastern/Latin American was not given a group of its own, so it appears it was lumped in with NZ European. Not that it makes a lot of difference considering the population spread.

Data obtained from the Ministry of Health survey for 2016-17 showed that in 2013, an estimated 598,000 people were identified as having depression. Whether this is an actual diagnosis or not is unclear. Based on these estimates, 13 per cent of New Zealanders were identified as having depression. That number increased in estimates each year in the report.

Table 2: **ESTIMATES BY ETHNICITY**

ETHNICITY WITH DEPRESSION	TOTAL	PERCENTAGE OF TOTAL POPULATION
NZ European/Other	492,000	11%
Maori	71,000	1.6%
Pacific	16,000	0.36%
Asian	19,000	0.4%

Table 3: **PERCENTAGE BY ETHNICITY**

Again, bear in mind that these are estimates. The percentages here are based on the total population of each ethnicity, not the total population as a whole.

ETHNICITY	PERCENTAGE
NZ European/Other	16%
Maori	11.9%
Pacific	5%
Asian	4%

When we look at the estimates for NZ European, it seems proportionate. However, when we look at the percentage of Maori, based on the number obtained in the Census, it seems disproportionate. There could be several reasons for this and I can make the following assumptions.

High numbers of Maori tend to live in poorer areas. Poverty, homelessness, smoking, drinking and chronic illness, such as diabetes, are also factors. As in the chapter on causes of depression, many of these are noted.

Around 20 per cent of New Zealand women were estimated in the 2016 Health Survey to have depression. The number is lower for men at 13 per cent. Further data can be reviewed online through the Ministry of Health website.

As depression is a major factor in death by suicide, it is necessary to look at some of the suicide statistics.

In 2018, a report was put together from a national Mental Health Enquiry. In the report, it was stated that New Zealand is among the worst in the OECD for suicide rates for young people. Of course, this impacts not just the family and friends, but the wider community as a whole.

There have been calls for investigations into some suicides, with some grieving families blaming a poor level of care in mental health. The lack of funding and poor resources has been a bone of contention for some time. While there have been moves to rectify this, we are yet to see how successful these efforts are.

An article in the *New Zealand Herald* in 2019 stated that the suicide rate in New Zealand is fairly high (Boyle, 2019).

According to the article, there were 668 suicides recorded in the 2017/18 year, with the rate at 13.67 per 100,000 population.

Of the total recorded, there were 142 suicides among the Maori population. Male Maori accounted for 97 of those.

While New Zealand's statistics appear to be higher, it should be noted that we have better access to health care, relatively speaking, than other countries. While not every family in New Zealand can afford GP visits, we are still in a better position than most. What this means for the numbers is that more people seek help for depression.

In a report published by the Mental Health Foundation in the UK, in 2013, depression was reported as the second leading cause of years lived with disability worldwide. The foundation also noted that depression was a major contributor in other health issues such as suicide and heart problems, which causes a heavy burden on the country's health system (Mental Health Foundation, 2016).

The report also included the following statistics:

- 19.7 per cent of people in the UK aged 16 and older showed symptoms of anxiety or depression.
- The numbers were higher among females at 22.5 per cent, while males were 16.8 per cent.

Nearly 6,000 suicides occurred in the UK in 2017, according to the foundation and it is considered to be the leading cause of death for those aged between 20 and 34. The numbers of men dying by suicide are around triple that of women. Those thought to be at the highest risk are men aged 40 to 44 years, where the rate is around 24 per 100,000 population..

The National Health Survey in Australia (Australian Bureau of Statistics, 2018) noted the following:

- Around one in 10 Australians reported depression or feelings of depression in 2017-18 or 10.4 per cent of the population. This was an increase from 2014-15, which was 8.9 per cent.

The data from the survey came from people who reported their condition as current and lasting six months or more.

A further breakdown of statistics was obtained from https://www.beyondblue.org.au/media/statistics.

- One in seven Australians are likely to experience depression within their lifetime.
- One in 16 are currently experiencing depression between the ages of 16 to 85.
- Women are more likely than men to experience depression, with an estimated one in six likely to experience depression in their lifetime compared to one in eight men.

The survey stated that 11.6 per cent of women

reported depression while the number of men was 9.1 per cent.

According to *Beyond Blue*, suicide accounts for a high proportion of deaths among those aged between 15 to 24 with suicide accounting for 36 per cent of deaths among those aged 15 to 24. In those aged 25 to 34, it was 30.9 per cent.

Death by suicide is more likely to occur in men rather than women. In statistics from 2016, of the Australians who died by suicide, 75 per cent of them were men and 25 per cent were women.

Statistics also show that indigenous people, i.e. Aboriginal and Torres Strait Islanders are more likely to die by suicide, with the death rate calculated at 25.5 per 100,000, compared to 12 per 100,000 for non-indigenous.

It begs the question: why are the numbers greater in certain areas?

The authors on Beyond Blue suggest that men were far less likely to seek help than women. The question is, why? Is it that they don't talk about it? Are they not wanting to be perceived as weak? Or perhaps they lack self-awareness?

If suicide rates are higher in men than women, then clearly something is not working.

In terms of the indigenous population, rates of psychological distress may be attributed to issues of racism, and low employment which affects their wellbeing.

Statistics from the National Institute for Mental Health in the United States paint a similar picture.

A survey on the prevalence of major depressive episodes conducted in 2017 survey estimated around 17.3 million adults in the United States had at least one major depressive episode. This represented 7.1 per cent of all American adults (over the age of 17).

Table 4 below shows the statistics by gender, age and ethnicity. Note the percentages are based on the percentage scores, rather than total population score.

The statistics for suicide rates by ethnicity paint a harsher picture (NIMH Mental Health Information statistics on suicide).

These statistics were supplied to the National Institute by the Center for Disease Control. In 2016, there were more than twice as many deaths by suicide as there were homicides in the United States, and the institute states it is the tenth leading cause of death overall.

TABLE 4: AMERICAN PREVALENCE OF DEPRESSION

Statistical Group	Percentage
Gender	
Male	5.30%
Female	8.70%

Age	
18-25	13.10%
26-49	7.70%
50+	4.7%

Ethnicity	
Hispanic	5.40%
White	7.90%
Black	5.40%
Asian	4.40%
Native Hawaiian/Other Pacific Islander	4.70%
Native American/Alaskan Native	8.00%

TABLE 5: SUICIDE RATES

Suicide Rates by Ethnicity per 100,000 population		
	Male	Female
Hispanic	11.6	2.8
White	26.5	7.9
Black	10.5	2.4
Asian/Pacific Islander	10.2	3.6
American Indian/Alaskan Native	32.8	10.2

I must point out that statistics cannot always be taken on face value. We must allow for minor variations in the data collected, especially in a Census, as some people may not include certain data for personal reasons or may not be included in the population count. I can only interpret the data given, and allowances need to be made for any erroneous interpretations.

A lack of systemic data in other countries can also make a difference in the numbers worldwide.

Information sourced from the World Health Organisation shows the prevalence of depression by region. These numbers were estimated and reported in 2017.

TABLE 6: CASES OF DEPRESSIVE DISORDER BY REGION (World Health Organisation, 2017)

	(millions)	Percentage
Africa	52.98	16
Eastern Mediterranean	29.19	9
European	40.27	12
Americas	48.16	15
South-East Asia	85.67	27
Western Pacific	66.21	21

An article printed in the *Washington Post* in 2013 by journalist Caitlin Dewey stated that researchers found depression is the second-most cause of disability around the world. The World Health Organisation estimated that more than 4 per cent of the world's population have been diagnosed with depression.

As of 2017, the world population was around 7.53 billion. If we take four per cent of that number, it adds up to just over 301 million. If the number is more than 4 per cent, that is still more than 300 million people worldwide with depression.

The important thing to note is that the percentage reached in the study was based on data already available. It does not account for the different variables, for example: that there are some countries with poor or no access to health care. Even in the United States, given that health care is expensive, many people would not have access to the type of care they need and may not be officially diagnosed.

What can be taken from the data is that in some areas, it would be expected to be higher, given the numbers of conflicts and constant violence, particularly in the Middle East.

Journalist Wana Udobang stated in an article published on Yahoo! Lifestyle in 2018 that the subject of mental health in Nigeria is still not discussed.

The country's Federal Neuro-Psychiatric Hospital estimates 21 million Nigerians have mental health issues, but this does not include another 30 million cases that go unreported.

Udobang states in her article that mental health issues are considered a 'Western' problem and it is difficult to seek treatment for depression. Those doing so are thought to be 'attention-seeking'.

Her article notes that of all the nations in the world, of which there are more than 180, Nigeria is ranked 30 in the list of the most suicide-prone, according to statistics from the World Health Organisation. While there are mental health services available, about one in 50 Nigerians seek help.

About 7 million people in Nigeria are estimated to be living with depression. If the above number is true, that is less than half a per cent of that estimate seeking help, which is staggering.

The World Health Organisation website also states that nearly 800,000 people per year die by suicide. Given this number, it is little wonder that depression is a major concern for such organisations.

Someone I know observed that depression does not appear to be as prevalent in third-world countries. I would have to question that. As the article above states, the perception is that depression is a Western problem, but is it? The point is, even if the statistics do not reflect it, that does not necessarily mean it does not exist in those areas. It may just mean that some people have never been correctly diagnosed.

There are obviously some barriers to those needing help for depression. Some of these would be cultural, while others would be a lack of resources, a lack of trained health-care providers and social stigma. It is also possible that it has been mis-diagnosed and that the problem may be something else entirely.

The statistics in this chapter only tell a small proportion of the story. Estimates seem to increase each year, but does that necessarily mean the problem is getting worse, or is it that more people are seeking help?

We will probably never know for sure.

Section Five: Managing Depression

The first thing to understand about managing depression is that it is about taking control of it, rather than letting it control you. It will not be easy initially. The second thing to understand about it is that you will have those days where things seem bad or outside forces in your life just seem to be conspiring against you.

The next thing is learning to recognise the early signs of a depressive episode and dealing with it or working through it, rather than letting it control you.

Above all, remind yourself that you are **not** alone, and you do not have to do this alone.

Depression is not a one size fits all illness. Everyone experiences it differently. The same is true for any kind of management strategy.

Robert Burton, in *The Anatomy of Melancholy* (1621) said that a healthy diet, enough sleep, music and 'meaningful work' could help combat 'melancholy'. However, Burton was writing in the 17th century, so while his ideas have not changed, the nature of them has.

We know more about depression now than we ever did. We know that it can be caused by a myriad of things and is not necessarily just a problem in the brain.

The way to manage depression is not only through medication. Everyone is different and may seek different methods to help them deal with it. In this section, I will explore some of the strategies and tools that anyone can use to help them.

These are just options. Ultimately, what you choose to take on board is your decision. Not everyone will be comfortable or will be able to use some of these strategies due to other pressures in their lives.

Chapter Thirty-Three: Natural

I came across an article from author and mental health advocate Therese Borchard and I thought I should address it from my perspective.

Therese's website lists her bio as Contributing Editor at *HealthCentral* and associate editor at *PsychCentral*, both American magazine/blogging type websites. She is also a founder of some online depression communities like **Group Beyond Blue**.

Therese's article: 9 Steps to Treat Depression Naturally (Borchard, 2015) was written for people who were not responding to conventional treatment. As someone who has been through it herself, she was writing from experience. She adds that she is still essentially a work-in-progress and still has her bad days. As we all do.

Firstly, she does not suggest that those on medication should just throw it away. I do not advocate this either.

1. Underlying Conditions

As you will have read already, some chronic conditions and some physiological conditions can be major factors in depression. It is important to get yourself checked.

Therese lists some illnesses like Crohn's Disease, hypothyroidism, low stomach acid, connective tissue problems, and vitamin deficiency.

I am a little cynical when it comes to the medical profession so take it with a grain of salt when I say that not all doctors will be willing to check for these things, and you should discuss any concerns with them. It is helpful to do a little reading on these as well. However, please do not rely on the Internet for all your answers.

I have had doctors in the past be dismissive of my concerns. In one instance, I had my thyroid checked and was told by my GP that it was fine, but a nutritionist felt otherwise, hence my cynicism.

2.   Eliminate Triggers of Inflammation

Therese notes some foods create inflammation in our brains. Some people may have sensitivities to certain types of foods, like gluten or sugar. This will be explored more in the nutrition chapter, but to use a pun, it's food for thought.

We are also exposed to toxins every day – from vehicle emissions and cigarette smoke to chemicals in the water we drink or swim in.

3.   Go Green

Try to eat a lot of green, leafy vegetables such as spinach, and kale as they provide a lot of nutrients.

4.   Heal Your Gut

This is another part that will be discussed in the nutrition chapter but there are theories that gut health plays a vital role in reducing the risk of depression.

5.   Yoga

While any kind of activity lifts your mood, Yoga is great because it can help with anxiety as well. When I have an anxiety attack, I start to hyperventilate, which causes me to tense up even more than I already am.

Yoga is more a gentle exercise but has an emphasis on breathing exercises and flexibility. Another good example of this kind of exercise is Tai Chi.

6. Reduce Stress

It is not as easy as it sounds. We all have busy lives, and for some, it might seem almost impossible. Especially if you are in a job where stress comes with the territory.

Financial stress is also a big one and if you are like thousands of others living below the bread line, it is not easy to get away from.

We all know when we are extremely stressed. Our heart rate goes up and we often feel like punching a wall.

Employ different strategies. If you are stressed by something at work, get up and walk away for five minutes, if at all possible. I am aware this is easier said than done. Even if you have to wait until your break, find a quiet place and practice deep breathing. This helps reduce any physiological issues caused by the stress.

If the stress is constant, especially in the job, consider changing jobs. Above all, your job is not worth sacrificing your health. Again, I am all too aware that this is easier said than done. Some countries have varying rules around paid labour. If you do find yourself in such a situation where conditions are detrimental to your health, I suggest talking to your local labour board to find out your rights.

7. Take Supplements

There are natural supplements available which can work with whatever other methods you are employing. However, some caution is needed. Please do not rely too heavily on these supplements and do some research. These tend to be quite expensive and should really only be taken to *supplement* your nutrition plan, not replace it.

It is always best to talk to a naturopath or a natural health professional who can advise you on what will work best and at what dose. Guesswork is not advised.

8.   Protect Your Sleep

It is one of the most important and probably the hardest of all to follow. Chronic sleep problems are one of the main characteristics of depression.

Try to get into a routine. Go to bed the same time every night and wake up at the same time every morning. Regardless of whether it is weekends or a weekday. I have read that trying to catch up on sleep on weekends or days off is not the best approach.

Seven to eight hours is usually recommended as the ideal length of time.

Turn off those electronic devices. According to scientists, using these devices right before sleep interferes with your internal clock, making it harder to fall asleep. If you have electronic devices such as an I-pad or a Kindle, health professionals recommend you turn those off at least 30 minutes before bed and either read books or do some other relaxing activity that doesn't involve using electronics.

There are also relaxation techniques you can try to help wind down.

9.   Find a Purpose

I was once talking to someone who talked about this very thing. I was in a job which was not fulfilling and was causing a lot of stress. He basically told me that if my heart was not in it, then do what was in my heart to do - of course this was writing.

We all need to have some sense of purpose. As I have alluded to elsewhere, writing, for me, proved to be a lifesaver. If I had not joined online fandoms and begun writing fan fiction, I feel very strongly that I would not still be here.

Others I have talked to agree on this approach. Things such as developing a hobby, finding a different job, focusing on self-care, or going for long walks are all ways they have found to be successful in helping them manage their depression.

Bear in mind that these are just some options and can be considered as stand-alone strategies or combined with others.

Chapter Thirty-Four: Therapy

Therapy has its origins in Greek history as a word for curing or healing a medical condition. Hydrotherapy, aromatherapy, hypnotherapy and psychotherapy all have similar aims.

In this chapter, I will explore some of the therapies available in managing depression.

Like anyone of my generation or younger, I am familiar with the Internet and some of the posts from various 'experts' claiming they have the answers to treating depression. They suggest that if we do 'such and such' we can change our whole outlook.

This is sometimes considered Pop Psychology.

Pop Psychology or Pseudo-Science

Pop Psychology, otherwise known as Popular Psychology, can be many things. They are mostly theories that appear to have some scientific basis but have little or no validity. By this, I mean that while the theory may claim to have some effect, positive or negative, on a person's illness, the conclusion is not based on any scientific evidence or tests. Hence it is invalid. It is also known as pseudo-science, whereby it is a fake science with no real proof of what it claims.

While I hesitate to use the phrase 'real psychology', the difference between pseudo-science theories and those by the likes of modern-day psychologists is what is known as empirical evidence. This is obtained through data collected by observation or experiments. However, it is not simply a matter of a researcher running an experiment and presenting their data. Their report has to be presented to the scientific community for what is called peer review. Their hypothesis is tested many times to ensure that their results are not a 'one-off'. If the results can be replicated successfully and sufficiently, the experiment is considered a success and any claims made from that report are validated.

Freud would be considered pop psychology nowadays, simply because his theories were untested. In his time, of course, those theories were just accepted, and anyone who questioned would claim it was too complex to be tested.

As in the chapter on causes of depression, there are several theories as to what really causes depression, and while they do sound plausible, my suggestion is to question everything. If there is actual evidence, whether, by observation or data, which proves that claim, we can take it to mean there is some validity. For instance, my own theories have been based on my own observations and some of the research I have done. However, it should be pointed out that there is also some observational bias. Someone else may come to a different conclusion based on their own observations of my behaviour. That is not to say that both conclusions are wrong as it is a matter of perspective.

Be careful of any posts on Facebook or any other type of social media which make claims that they can 'cure' depression. Ask yourself questions: do they have evidence to back up their claims? Are they able to be tested? Is there any scientific basis to these claims, or are they just based on the poster's personal experience? In other words, check out these claims but view them with a certain sense of scepticism.

Affirmations

Author Louise Hay is probably one of the first to use a technique called affirmations.

According to her website, she had a harsh upbringing and as a teenager, ended up in New York City where she became a model, then married a prominent businessman. Following the breakup of her marriage, she trained as a minister in the Church of Religious Science. She began counselling clients and developed her philosophy of creating health through positive thought patterns.

Her reference guide, *Heal Your Body*, was a compilation of positive thoughts and released in the mid-1970s. She went on to publish *You Can Heal Your Life* in 1984. She collaborated with others to publish more books and DVDs.

Louise's method was to use positive affirmations by looking at your reflection in the mirror and saying something such as: *I now free myself from destructive fears and doubts.*

I did read Louise's book several years ago, but her method of affirmation was something that I was not comfortable with. However, there is nothing to say someone else cannot try it for themselves.

Bear in mind, however, that this is more likely based on a religious philosophy than a scientific one.

Law of Attraction

There have been many theories concerning the Law of Attraction which have become extremely popular. The premise of these theories is essentially the ability to draw into our lives what we are focusing on.

So, if you need money, you focus and, eventually, the 'universe' will provide.

However, there is one thing that is rarely pointed out and I think should be questioned when considering this approach. That is the idea that, if something negative has happened to you, the law of attraction implies that you have somehow sent out that negative message and it has come back to you.

It sounds to me very similar to the general law of physics.

Every action has an equal and opposite reaction. Many religions also use this philosophy in the sense that what you put out is returned to you in some way. Some would call it karma.

Physician and researcher, Dr Neil Farber wrote in a blog in *Psychology Today* that the law of attraction does not exist.

He stated that, rather than being based on scientific theory, it was pseudoscience, based on unfounded and erroneous assumptions.

In some theories on the law of attraction, it is often suggested to live life as if you already have the things you want, which is logically impossible. Take, for instance, wealth. If we lived as if we already had an abundance of money available to us, we would soon end up in serious trouble, not only financially but also legally.

Most people would create goals and plans in order to figure out their life direction. Yet in some of these theories, it feels as if I am being led to believe that such things are unnecessary.

Take, for example, the idea that an athlete is told to visualise performing in their particular sport. They visualise so much that they see themselves actually not only reaching their personal goal but winning. However, do you think they would do this without training? Visualisations are great at helping someone focus on their ultimate goal, but they don't help them get there. Only training can do that.

Of course, the suggestion that anyone can just achieve such things without hard work is ridiculous, and there is no suggestion in what research is available on the Law of Attraction that it does happen this way, but it can easily be perceived so.

Dr Farber also notes that when negative things happen, by the law of attraction, it is always 'our fault'. That somehow we were thinking bad things. It is a faulty premise that is fundamental to the Law of Attraction and one of the things that bothers me the most about it.

Let's take, for example, cancer. By this premise, anyone who gets cancer does so because they 'attract' it. By the same token, depression happens because we are thinking about it and attract it to us. Huh?

Having watched my father waste away from cancer, having watched others go through it, why would anyone want to attract it? This is why this idea bothers me so much. Maybe that is not what most people mean when they talk about the Law of Attraction, but this is how I perceive it.

The point is, no amount of wishing and visualising will give us what we want without hard work. After all, with all the years I have visualised myself winning the lottery, by that token, I would have won the big prize many times over.

There is nothing wrong with positive visualisations as long as there is an awareness that it is not something that comes to you by magic.

There are those who believe in the 'law of attraction' and that the above is too negative a view. That is fine. My suggestion is to be open-minded but also try to be objective when reading such theories. My intention was only to point out some inconsistencies. The simple truth is that, to the best of my knowledge, there is no empirical evidence which proves the existence of the law of attraction or that it actually works.

Talk Therapies

First, there are differences between a counsellor, psychologist and a psychiatrist.

A counsellor is required to have a level 7 Bachelor's Degree. More information on this can be found on the NZQA website.

They also need skills in counselling and knowledge of different theories and techniques, research, communication and listening skills, an understanding of human development and relationships, knowledge of social and cultural issues and knowledge of self-care strategies. To become a provisional member of the New Zealand Association of Counsellors, they also need 200 hours of supervised clinical practice. Check out the NZ

Association of Counsellors website, or local websites if you are outside of New Zealand.

A registered psychologist has studied the field for many years and draws on scientific research to provide effective treatment. In New Zealand, they must have at least a Master's degree in psychology, have at least 1500 hours of accredited practical training and be registered with the New Zealand Psychologists Board. They must also have a current Annual Practising Certificate. For Kiwis, check the Ministry of Business and Innovation for more information on this.

In New Zealand, a psychiatrist must first complete the Health Sciences Programme at Otago University, or the first year of the Bachelor of Health Sciences or Bachelor of Science in Biomedical Science, then complete a five year Bachelor of Medicine and Bachelor of Surgery degree, work for one to two years as a junior doctor in a hospital before completing another five years of training through the Royal Australian and New Zealand College of Psychiatrists Fellowship programme (Careers website: Psychiatrist).

A psychiatrist has the ability to prescribe medication. The other two do not.

For years I had gone to see counsellors, and while their suggested strategies appeared to help for a while, I would soon find myself going back down again. It bothered me that their strategies did not seem to 'stick'.

The ultimate goal for counselling is to have help to manage whatever you are feeling so that you can get to a point where you can manage without that help.

At times I would get so annoyed with myself for not being able to take whatever the counsellor said on board. Then I found someone who has been able to do what other counsellors have not. Help me get to that point.

The important thing with a counsellor or therapist is that they have to be able to understand who you are and your thought processes. It is not an easy thing to do. Some may follow specific theories, like cognitive behavioural therapy (CBT), while others will merely be a guide to your own self-healing process.

As I have learnt, it is not a simple matter of visiting one counsellor. Sometimes it is trial and error to find the right one. I have been extremely lucky to have found someone who is not only very good at what they do, but also 'gets me' and helps me discover things for myself.

For instance, I have had several counsellors tell me, in the past, I needed to 'let go' of my anger toward my father for the way I was brought up. When I would ask them how I'm supposed to do that, I would never get a clear answer. I did not have the tools to do so, and no one seemed to want to provide me with them. Until I began working with my last counsellor.

I have had sessions with someone who has made me feel uncomfortable talking about what I have gone through. Talking is not easy, and it's worse when you do not trust your therapist. You are lucky if you find someone who is non-judgemental. I am not saying counsellors are meant to be impartial. Sometimes it helps if they relate to you on some level so they can be an advocate for you if necessary.

Talking with a psychiatrist or counsellor is not always how it looks on television. There is not always a leather couch where you can lay down and talk about your day. Nor is there a therapist sitting in an armchair with a notepad listening to you talk and answering with a 'hmm, and how do you feel about that?' Personally, that would irritate me to no end.

The one thing I have noticed about therapy is the way the rooms are set up. I have already mentioned the short online course through King's College and it was interesting to see that much emphasis was placed on how the therapist or psychologist is situated in terms of their patient. Like sitting facing the patient may lead them to feel uncomfortable, and in some cases, intimidated. Suggestions are made like sitting at right angles to the patient, so the space is more 'open', giving them less of a feeling of being 'trapped'.

A counsellor's demeanour may also help. If they are friendly and open, rather than combative, this can also play a huge part in how they relate to the patient/client. The one thing that may help in this instance is knowing whether they can 'walk a mile in your shoes'. If they have some experience or knowledge of what you have gone through, either through their own experience or through a family member, it helps. This does not necessarily mean they have had depression. They may have experienced certain stressors, which in turn allows them to understand what you have gone through.

I must emphasise that you must be able to feel you can trust your counsellor. This has nothing to do with ethics. You are basically sharing your innermost thoughts and feelings, and sometimes a few secrets. While your counsellor is bound by certain laws regarding patient confidentiality, it goes much deeper than that. Again, it is about them being non-judgemental and allowing you to feel that you can share this information without fear that they will use that information against you.

One of the counsellors I went to, and one of the reasons I stopped going to them, was because they told me I blamed everyone else for my issues. While there is an element of personal responsibility, I know my depression stems from something that I did not cause myself. I had to learn to get past that before I could begin to explore my personal responsibility.

There are qualified counsellors who can help you with your journey. Their methods may vary, but an important part of counselling is to come to an understanding of where the depression comes from and how to manage it.

Counselling is just one aspect of psychotherapy which encompasses a number of different theoretical practices. These practices include cognitive behavioural therapy, mindfulness-based cognitive therapy and psychodynamic theory.

There is also traditional Freudian psychotherapy which focuses on childhood traumas as the root cause.

Cognitive Behavioural Therapy (CBT)

Cognitive behavioural therapy centres around behaviour and modifying that behaviour. For instance, in my own case, my behaviours around my perception of self-image. CBT would identify the thoughts driving that perception and work on modifying those behaviours and try to alter my perception.

CBT has its roots in therapies developed in the 1970s. Behavioural therapists theorised that certain behaviours were due to more than just environmental factors.

In a textbook on Psychology, the authors suggest that cognitive behavioural therapists focus less on what Freud was interested in, i.e. painful events in the client's past, and more on changing the way the patient behaved in the present (Carlson & Buskist, 1997).

In terms of depression, American psychiatrist Aaron Beck developed a theory where negative beliefs were based on faulty logic. Once the fault is recognised, the therapy explores ways to correct the perception, thus correcting the behaviour.

This kind of therapy has been criticised by more 'traditional' therapists because it focuses on the symptom of psychological problems but excludes root causes.

While many problems of depression can stem from things that occurred in the past, those who advocate CBT believe it is possible to change behaviours without delving into those events (Carlson & Buskist, 1997).

In some cases, CBT focuses on negative thinking patterns and gets the patient to think about the same thing in another way. For instance, my considering myself a failure because I'm not rich or do not have my own home. CBT would discourage that kind of black and white thinking and encourage me to focus on what I have achieved. It's rather a generalisation but it is the best example I can come up with.

The effectiveness of CBT can only be evaluated through experiments. One such evaluation was reported in an article published in 2016 (Brown, et al, 2016).

The authors were looking at a training program implemented by the Veterans Health Administration. This was a national initiative in response to a concern over the numbers of veterans dying by suicide in the United States.

The program included workshop training on using CBT to treat depression.

More than 900 veterans participated in the program with varying levels of depression and/or suicidal ideations. By the end of the program, the results did show some reduction in depression and the authors note the results were consistent with other studies.

However, they also noted some limitations: firstly, that the findings were from patients who received treatment as part of the training program. They felt more evaluation from previously trained CBT therapists might have given stronger results. Secondly, that it was an evaluation of the program, rather than a controlled trial.

Psycho-Dynamic Theory

The term is rooted in the studies of Sigmund Freud. While it was believed that rational, conscious processes governed behaviour, the Austrian psychotherapist saw it somewhat differently in that there were various conflicts between such things as instinct and reason in the brain (Carlson & Buskist, 1997).

Freud, (1856-1939) trained in neurology in the lab of physiologist and neuroanatomist, Ernst Wilhelm von Brückle. It was through his work there that he would later adopt his method of making detailed observations about his patients.

Following this, he studied under neurologist Jean-Martin Charcot, in Paris. Charcot's work with patients with hysteria also became the basis of some of Freud's theories. Hysteria was a term used to describe a psychological disorder where a patient's psychological stress would become physiological symptoms. If you have ever seen the '70s Korean war black comedy *M*A*S*H*, there is an episode in which a patient appears to be paralysed, but the doctors can find no physiological reason and determine it is hysterical paralysis (*Mad Dogs and Servicemen*, 1974).

Charcot believed that psychological trauma was behind the hysteria, and this was explored in the *M*A*S*H* episode - the patient was the sole survivor of a slaughter in the Korean War.

Freud's studies led him to form the theory that past trauma was the reason for various psychological issues.

In connection with therapy for depression, it is exploring past issues and events in an attempt to discover the root causes. This may be dealing with traumatic events or something else.

This is not always a popular type of therapy, particularly with friends and family. They might suggest you are 'dwelling too much in the past' and want you to move on. However, for some, they may be ignoring the past at the expense of their present. It isn't as simple as it sounds when you have years of negative self-talk behind you. In order to let go, you need to be able to identify where the negative self-talk comes from.

For instance, my own feelings about my father. I could not move on from my feelings of anger until I dealt with it.

It is the same as some physical ailments. Would you heal a broken leg by telling yourself you don't need to dwell on how you broke your leg? No. You would still have to heal the break. You would need to remind yourself how the incident occurred in the first place so in future you will be more careful.

You cannot heal yourself if you do not know what caused the wound in the first place. Otherwise, you are just treating symptoms. In my case, since my father was part of the problem, I had to stop blaming him and see him from a different perspective.

Counselling helped me do that. I learnt to see things from his perspective, and it brought me to an understanding of why he did the things he did. No one else had ever approached it in that way before, and it was as if a lightbulb had suddenly switched on over my head.

I have since applied the same theory in other areas of my past with a great deal of success.

As with any kind of treatment, there are pros and cons. One of the major cons of therapy is a general perception that anyone who tries therapy has some serious psychological problems.

This could not be further from the truth. Put it this way: we go to a doctor when we are feeling unwell. There is no stigma attached to this. So why should there be such a stigma attached to getting any kind of psychotherapy?

Taking the step to therapy is not an easy one, and some outside influences might even try to talk you out of it.

It can also be costly. Most people who are working do not have the financial help to pay for sessions, and the cost can range from as little as $50 to hundreds of dollars per session. There may be ways around this, depending on where in the world you are and what options are available. Check with your healthcare provider.

Some pros:

1.   Counsellors have the training to deal with all manner of issues. No subject is taboo.

Coupled with that, counsellors are bound by a Code of Ethics. There is a website you can visit for further information. This is listed at the end of the book.

2.   Talking things through helps you see things from a different perspective. Having a neutral party also helps.

The counsellor's only interest is in helping you work through your issues.

By talking over things with a counsellor, it may help you to understand more about what caused the depression and how to deal with it.

3.   Letting out pent-up emotions helps you deal with them.

We all tend to suppress our emotions, and it can create conflict in families. Being able to express those emotions in a safe environment helps avoid that conflict.

4.   It gives you time out to confront your issues.

Work, family, or other activities do not give you time to think about what is going on in your life, and can add to your stress, so there are times when you really do need to give yourself some space to work things through. By spending time with a counsellor, it's allowing that time.

6.   It helps to know you are not alone.

The worst thing about depression is the feeling that you are on your own. No matter how supportive a family member is, they cannot really understand what you are going through. Sometimes a counsellor who has been through it themselves makes it easier to relate.

7.   The adage of a problem shared is a problem halved.

As above, talking about those pent-up feelings makes it easier to deal with them.

8.   It may help you to become more aware of when you are having a depressive episode, and what caused it, thus you are able to deal with it more easily.

A counsellor can teach you strategies so that when you are having an episode of depression or anxiety, you can implement those strategies, lessening the severity of the episode.

9.   It helps improve your physical wellbeing.

It's well-known that stress is a factor in many physical ailments. If talking through things helps ease the stress, it will help in other ways.

Understandably, not everyone is keen to try therapy. It can take a lot of false starts, a lot of trial and error to find someone who is the right fit for you, or you may decide not to use it at all.

Chapter Thirty-Five: Being Active

With all the research in the field of mental health, experts are now finding that a more holistic approach is an important part of treating illnesses like depression.

Health professionals know there is a link between chronic health problems and depression. These can be anything from diabetes to heart problems. Chronic pain can be very wearing on a patient, and it's not difficult to understand why this leads to depression. Doctors often advocate exercise as a way of combatting those problems. But what if the depression is not caused by chronic health problems? Should the same rule apply?

In a word, yes.

Experts agree that physical activity is highly beneficial to our physical health, but it also helps reduce the risk of developing depressive episodes. There are several reasons:

1. It provides structure
2. It helps connect us with nature
3. Positive engagement with others
4. We sleep better

When we talk about exercise, the first thing that probably comes to mind is working out in a gym. Of beefy guys lifting massive weights, or skinny women running on treadmills.

Most health professionals suggest working out for around 30 minutes a day at least three to four times a week, or more if possible. Some suggest around 150 minutes, or 30 minutes five times a week.

But what should that exercise consist of? Jogging? Swimming? Lifting weights?

Actually, it can be any of those things, or it could be something just as simple as walking.

In my own experience, while trying to lose weight for a major operation, I began walking around Hamilton, where I was living at the time. I was also doing my best to stay away from various junk foods.

I started off slowly by walking around the campus at Waikato University. They had a walking track which bordered a playing field. Some of it would lead into the campus itself, but I would walk just the main one which was around two kilometres. As my fitness improved, I increased the distance until I was walking up to five kilometres a day.

The first thing I noticed was that I began sleeping a little better. Then, as I lost weight, I began feeling fitter, and my moods were more stable. I was still having moments of stress, but these were mostly of my own making, as I was working on a new novel at the time and trying to get it edited and published and I was working odd hours. Still, my response to the stress was more manageable.

Now I find when I go out walking or cycling, it has a way of 'clearing the cobwebs' and making me feel better in myself. Part of it, of course, is pride that I have done something good for myself, but, as the professionals I have talked to suggest, it is also due to a release of hormones.

In a TED talk, neuroscientist Wendy Suzuki (quoted with permission from TED talks) discusses the benefits of exercise on the brain. The benefits in terms of depression will be discussed in more detail later. However, Wendy's talk also mentions currently incurable diseases like Alzheimer's.

"The most transformative thing that exercise will do is its protective effects on your brain. Here you can think about the brain like a muscle. The more you're working out, the bigger and stronger your hippocampus and prefrontal cortex gets. Why is that important? Because the prefrontal cortex and the hippocampus are the two areas that are most susceptible to neurodegenerative diseases and normal cognitive decline in aging."

To put it another way, you might still be susceptible to Alzheimer's Disease, but the exercise will help slow the progress of the disease.

In the chapter on causes, I cited an article in which researchers noted the hippocampus was smaller in patients with depression. While I must reiterate the results are open to interpretation, given Dr Suzuki's assertions on the positive effects of exercise on the brain, it goes without saying that being active can help someone with depression.

Dr Sarah Gingell expands further on this in a blog in Psychology Today.

"Evidence is accumulating that many mental health conditions are associated with reduced neurogenesis in the hippocampus. The evidence is particularly strong for depression." (quoted with permission, Gingell, 2018)

Neurogenesis is defined as the growth of nerve tissue.

We know that the hippocampus is a region of the brain that affects memory. Dr Gingell suggests that when we have mental health issues, our brain is unable to adapt to new or unexpected conditions. She calls it cognitive inflexibility, and it simply means we continue with behaviours that basically are unhealthy and do little to help our depression. "It is therefore plausible that exercise leads to better mental health in general, through its effects on systems that increase the capacity for mental flexibility (Gingell, 2018).

Doctors in the UK also advocate physical activity. This does not necessarily mean signing up at a gym and working out for an hour. In fact, they say just ten minutes of physical activity can be just as beneficial as therapy or medication.

What Does Exercise Do?

We all know a sedentary lifestyle is bad for our health. Experts suggest it contributes to risk factors for obesity, cardiovascular disease and diabetes, but it also puts people at risk of developing mental health disorders, especially depression.

When we are less active, our metabolism slows. This in turn affects the body's ability to process things such as sugar and fat (Kandola, 2018). Most research on diet and exercise talks about how too much sugar and fat can accumulate in the body when we do not exercise adequately or eat the wrong things. Of course, there is much more to it than that.

Health experts are now claiming that a sedentary lifestyle and too much sugar has replaced smoking as the biggest health issue of our time.

When we feel depressed, we turn to things that, for a little while, help us feel better. This could be caffeine or junk food, for example. Caffeine can increase heart rate and blood pressure. Too much of it is obviously not a good thing and stopping it can create withdrawal symptoms like headaches. I have experienced this myself, when I stopped drinking coffee for a month. For over a week, I had pounding headaches.

We seek out comfort foods, like chocolate, sweets or various sweet pastries without really understanding why it is a comfort food. The problem is that, as we now know, sugar is not always good for our health.

Too much junk food causes weight gain, cholesterol, fatty tissue and of course, alcohol and drugs can inhibit brain function, among other troubles.

One factor most of the above all have in common is what is called endorphins. These are the body's 'feel-good messengers' and are the most well-known of all the neuro-transmitters. These are said to act like analgesics (pain-killers).

What does this have to do with exercise? You can get the same kind of 'good feelings' by exercising instead of these addictions.

For myself, if I am not working hard at the gym, I enjoy going for walks, doing what I call 'clearing out the cobwebs'.

Picture this: you're walking into an old shed or a cottage that hasn't been used in a while. Everywhere you look, you see dust and cobwebs. It's dark and smells a little musty. So you open the windows and the doors to let in some fresh air and clear the cobwebs and dust from the glass to let in the light.

Experts say that a similar thing happens when we exercise. In order to release stored energy, our muscles require oxygen. That's why our heart rate increases, and we feel breathless when we do any kind of strenuous activity.

Eventually, the body adjusts, and everything begins to equalise. This leads to a release of neurotransmitters, and we begin to feel good. Moods begin to stabilise, and we're happier. Ever feel that rush of adrenaline after a hard workout? That's those neurotransmitters releasing chemicals in the body.

Exercise allows us to control the depression, instead of it controlling us. Not everyone wants to use medication, and in some cases, the medication may make us feel 'out of it', or as Michelle put it, numb.

There is another benefit to exercise. Dr Gingell says it gives us a break from "current concerns and damaging self-talk" (Gingell, 2018).

Researchers conducted a study between 1998 and 2001 (Dunn et al., 2004) where participants were asked to undertake an exercise regimen. The participants were randomly split into groups and the amount of exercise each group did varied between the amount of energy expended to the frequency of exercise. Participants were aged between 20 and 45 years with mild to moderate depressive disorder.

For instance, some were required to do light exercise, while others were told to follow public health guidelines on exercise (for example: thirty minutes a day, five times a week).

What the study found was that exercise can help alleviate

symptoms of depression, but only after expending a certain amount of energy as prescribed by health experts. Light exercise did little to help.

In my own perspective, I feel a sense of accomplishment when I exercise. Whether I'm just out walking or going to the gym to do a hard workout, even though I'm ending up sweating and a little sore, I know I have done something good for myself.

Not everyone can afford to go to the gym or hire a personal trainer. However, it doesn't have to be working out at the gym. It can be anything from walking, running or swimming to gymnastics, or even dancing. Most experts recommend around thirty minutes a day. Choose whatever works for you.

Depression and anxiety can be overwhelming, and it's easy to use it as an excuse not to get off the couch to start any exercise routine. The best thing to do is start off small, with a walk around a local park or something similar. This was basically what I did when I started my weight-loss journey pre-surgery. I slowly built up to a distance I could tolerate without getting too tired.

Choose a good time of day when you're not busy with work or the family. Take the time to have your own space and be 'one with yourself'. Eventually, when you have gained some confidence and got into a routine, then you can try new things like going for a run, training with a friend or going to a gym or group fitness class.

As the ad says, it won't happen overnight, but it will happen. You won't start to feel better overnight, or in a week. If you are looking to lose weight, you won't lose tons of weight in a month. Even a little bit of exercise is still a positive step toward managing your depression.

The point is, be realistic. It's great if you have a goal in mind. Set mini-goals if it helps. If you start off thinking you are going to run a half-marathon in your first week, you are setting the bar too high. Above all, reward yourself when you reach that first target and keep going.

Chapter Thirty-Six: Eating Well

"Let food be thy medicine and let medicine be thy food," is a quote often attributed to Greek physician, Hippocrates. Research suggests that the man known as the 'father of medicine', who lived around 4th century BC, did not actually say this. However, it is a principle that would certainly fit with his teachings.

Regardless of whether he said it or not, it is clear nutrition plays an important role in treating illness.

I am not about to suggest that Hippocrates' philosophy of treating any illness with food or herbs will be a miracle cure. Far from it. The one thing that should be immediately clear is that the world of two thousand years ago is a far, far different world than the one we have today. It is well-known that the foods we eat bear little resemblance to those of ancient times and we have various factors to thank for that. For instance, environmental factors, genetic modifications, how food is stored, and so on.

Here's an example: a farmer who grows organic crops. It takes a few years before a farm can actually be certified. The problem is, how can we trust that his produce is truly organic if just a kilometre or so away, another farmer is using chemical pesticides or fertilisers?

'Diet' has become the buzzword for the 21st century. We've all heard about various diets, from Atkins, to South Beach, to paleo and plant-based diets. The first thing I would suggest is: ban the word 'diet'. For some, that word has negative connotations, so avoid it if possible. Instead, try to refer to it as a nutrition plan.

The second thing I would suggest is: read everything you can on various eating plans but don't take everything as gospel. Take notes and compare the differences, then decide what works for you.

Everyone's body works differently. Just because two people have depression doesn't mean that eating the same foods will help them in the same way. Perhaps one of them has diabetes, or Coeliac Disease. So, while one person must monitor their blood sugar, another must avoid gluten. While a gluten-free nutrition plan might work for the Coeliac it is not necessarily the right way to help them manage their depression.

The one thing most people never think about when it comes to what they eat is how it can affect their mood. Having had poor nutrition and eating habits most of my life, I can safely say there is a definite link. At my lowest point, I crave chocolate. Most of us know that chocolate can release various neuro-transmitters in the brain, like endorphins, or Phenylethylamine, otherwise known as the love drug. Some women tend to crave chocolate around their 'time of the month', whereby the hormones are pretty much going crazy.

I have also craved salty snacks (I go nuts for salt and vinegar potato chips, even if they are not necessarily good for my digestive system or my weight) at certain times, although I have noticed I crave them more if I'm feeling a bit down.

I do know that the more depressed I feel, the less likely I am to think about what I'm eating, and I make poor choices. Like another person with depression might turn to alcohol or drugs, I eat junk food. Which then becomes a vicious circle.

I can only assume that the temporary comfort I get from such things provides the right kind of chemical response. It probably goes without saying that when I eat a lot of junk food, it has both positive and negative results. Positive in that I perceive myself as feeling less low, but negative in that it means a late night as my stomach struggles to digest what I've eaten.

As I mentioned in an earlier chapter, I have always had a problem with vegetables. When I was younger, my reactions were akin to that of someone who had a phobia. I could not even look at a vegetable without feeling anxiety.

A few months ago, my counsellor tried an experiment. She had brought some cauliflower, a vegetable that I still hate to this day and would never eat and asked me to hold a piece of it. The smell reminded me of days when my father would cook vegetables and boil them so long there would be no goodness left in them. The smell would fill the kitchen and I would have to leave the room so I wouldn't get nauseous.

I sat down at the table in the kitchen of the house where I would meet my counsellor and held a piece of this thing in my hand. I felt its texture. Cauliflower looks rather weird, and in some ways, reminds me of the shape of a brain, even though it looks like a tree. It feels just as weird.

Yet, as I rolled it in my hand, I felt no anxiety. It was just a vegetable. However, the thought of cooking that up and eating it makes my stomach churn.

I have been able to eat some salads. However, because I am on a very tight budget, the cost of the ingredients are too expensive for me to justify spending so much money for it to only last a couple of days, so I rarely eat them. When I do, however, I do not have as many problems with them as I did when I was a child. The textures are still strange, but I can at least keep them down.

When I changed what I was eating, consuming fewer snacks and sweets, I not only lost weight, but I also felt better in myself. I do admit some of that was pride, because I had managed to beat those cravings back and I was starting to see positive changes in my body in a physiological sense. Trust me that when you hate what you see in the mirror, any change in image is for the better.

I have had terrible episodes of feeling stressed in the past, but when I eat foods rich in fatty acids like Omega-3 and Omega-6, I notice my stress levels are lower. I also feel my head is clearer. By that I don't just mean fewer migraines, but less 'fuzziness'. These fatty acids can usually be found in oily fish, like salmon and sardines. Don't like sardines? Try them on toast with baby spinach leaves. Okay, I use a lot of malt vinegar on mine, but I love sardines!

Articles I have researched confirm there is a lot of study going on that investigates the link between nutritional factors and human cognition, behaviour and emotions. While the causes of depression are still heavily debated, nutritional neuro-scientists have studied this quite extensively. According to one article, common mental disorders can be found in countries where dietary intake is deficient in many nutrients. For example, omega-3 fatty acids. (Sathyanarayana Rao, et al., 2008)

Using supplements of these vital nutrients also help reduce symptoms of depression, but, as in the earlier chapter, supplements should not be used as a replacement for the natural product.

Carbohydrates

Much maligned, carbohydrates are an essential part of nutrition. Research has shown that carbohydrates play an important role in the structure and function of an organism, including affecting mood and behaviour (Sathyanarayana Rao, et al., 2008). Yet, many diet plans persist in the idea that carbs are bad, and in some cases, should be eliminated.

Not all carbs are bad. According to the article authors cited above, a meal rich in carbohydrates triggers the release of insulin in the body, which lets blood sugar into the cells. In other words, carbs are necessary for energy. The question is, what carbs?

Experts suggest carbohydrates that are low on the Glycaemic Index are more useful as they are slower-acting which also means the effects last longer. A guide to these foods will be at the end of the chapter.

A good eating plan should also be rich in proteins as these

contain amino acids, which are the main building blocks. Foods rich in protein include meats, milk and other dairy products, and eggs.

Some nutrition plans advocate a plant-based diet. However, some experts still caution against such things, saying plant proteins may lack one or two amino acids. I have heard that it is possible to get these essential nutrients from plant-based foods as well. It is just a matter of knowing which ones.

In any case, it is important to do some careful research and even talk with a nutritionist to find out what is best for you.

One of the problems some of us face is the fact that we simply cannot afford to eat healthy. Which puts us between a rock and a hard place. Having been on a benefit, I am well aware there are not enough funds to afford some of the foods that nutritionists recommend. I cannot advise on this as I do not know a way around this myself. While on a benefit, my budget left me with barely $20 a week to cover food once everything else was paid. Not even a budget adviser can find a way around this.

Eating the right foods can be very expensive and it is little wonder many people find themselves eating bread or cheap foods most of the time. Sadly, the powers-that-be can be very short-sighted when it comes to providing enough for people to live on. I realise the benefit is only supposed to be a temporary measure, but in some circumstances, it can be difficult to get off it.

Research study

A team of researchers from around the world conducted a meta-analysis of studies into the link between nutrition and depression.

At the time of publication, the article stated that it was the only known meta-analysis of its type. Sixteen independent studies were analysed. However, they note that only one of those trials involved subjects diagnosed with clinical depression. "All the remaining 15 studies investigating effects of dietary interventions on symptoms of depression (were) in nonclinical depression samples." (Firth, et al., 2019, used with permission)

In an article published on the Western Sydney University website, the results noted from the study included a small but significant effect on reducing depressive symptoms.

However, female-only samples showed a significant difference whereas there was no significant difference in men.

Dr Joseph Firth, Senior Research Fellow at NICM Health Research Institute stated in the article that adopting better nutrition can boost mood, but further research would be required for clinically-diagnosed psychiatric disorders (Firth, 2019).

What the study is essentially saying is that good nutrition is a factor in managing depression. It does not necessarily help with symptoms of clinical depression, but that is less a fault of the concept and more a fault of the absence of sufficient studies focusing on the effects of nutrition on clinical depression.

Probiotics

There are theories now that gut health also has an effect on mood disorders. Dr Sandra Cabot mentions this in her book, *The Liver Cleansing Diet*.

If we think about it, the idea is very logical. If our gut health is poor, it stands to reason that it will have a flow-on effect to other parts of the body. Poor digestion can cause problems in organs like the kidneys or the liver. The brain is another organ, so why wouldn't bad digestion affect the brain as well?

Canadian health and science journalist and researcher Jordan Fallis wrote of his own struggles with stress and anxiety. In a blog on healthyholisticliving.com, he states that when he learnt of the gut-brain connection, he began taking probiotics.

However, he is careful to emphasise that probiotics alone will not be enough. "I also had to make changes to my diet, take key supplements, improve thyroid health and overcome trauma. There really is no quick fix or magic bullet." (Fallis, 2017, used with permission)

Jordan lists five probiotic strains which may be helpful:
1. Lactobacillus rhamnosus
2. Bifidobacterium longum
3. Lactobacillus reuteri
4. Lactobacillus fermentum
5. Bifidobacterium breve

Talk with your local health food store or your nutritionist to see if these are available in your area.

Plant-Based Diet

Contrary to popular belief, while the plant-based diet does advocate eating mostly foods derived from plants, it is not a completely vegan nutritional plan. However, it does suggest that your eating plan be made up primarily of plants, including: fruits, vegetables, nuts, seeds, legumes, beans and oils. You can still eat meat and poultry, but not as much.

Dietitian Katherine McManus wrote on Harvard Health Publishing that there have been studies on the Mediterranean Diet and a vegetarian diet.

According to the Mayo Clinic, the Mediterranean Diet consists of: vegetables, fruits, whole grains and healthy fats daily, fish, beans, poultry and eggs weekly, dairy products in moderation and limited red meat.

McManus (Harvard, 2019) states that this eating plan has been known to reduce risks of heart disease, metabolic syndrome, diabetes, some cancers, depression and improve mental and physical functions.

Vegetarian diets are also known to support health.

To help you out, here is a list of recommended foods and what they're best for:

Essential Fatty Acids – Brain Food

Omega 3 – Linolenic Acid
- Cold water high-fat fish like salmon, sardines, anchovies, mackerel, herring, trout

- Flaxseeds (oil, seeds, meal), hempseeds (oil, seeds), walnuts, pumpkin seeds, Brazil nuts, sesame seeds
- Avocados
- Dark green leafy vegetables like kale, spinach, mustard greens and collards

Omega 6 – Linoleic Acid
- Flaxseeds (oil, seeds, meal)
- Hempseed (oil, seeds)
- Grapeseed oil
- Pumpkin seeds, sunflower seeds
- Nuts (pignolia/pine, pistachios)
- Borage oil, evening primrose oil, blackcurrant seed oil
- Acai

Omega 9 – Oleic Acid
- Extra virgin olive oil
- Olives
- Avocados
- Nuts (almonds, peanuts, pecans, cashews, pistachios, hazelnuts, macadamias)
- Sesame oil

Glycaemic Index
Low GI (Range 55 or less)
- Fructose
- Beans (black, pinto, kidney, lentil, peanut, chickpea)
- Small seeds (sunflower, flax, pumpkin, poppy, sesame, hemp)
- Walnuts
- Cashews
- Most whole intact grains (durum, spelt, kamut)
- Wheat
- Millet
- Oat

- Rice
- Barley
- Most vegetables
- Most sweet fruits (peaches, strawberries, mangoes)
- Mushrooms
- Chillies

Medium GI (56-69)

- White sugar or sucrose
- Not intact whole wheat or enriched wheat
- Pita bread
- Basmati rice
- Unpeeled boiled potato
- Grape juice
- Raisins
- Prunes
- Pumpernickel bread
- Cranberry juice
- Regular ice cream
- Banana
- Sweet potato

High GI (70 and above)

- Glucose (dextrose, grape sugar)
- High fructose corn syrup
- White bread
- Most white rice
- Corn flakes
- Extruded breakfast cereals
- Maltose
- Maltodextrins
- White potato

The last thing I would advise is, consult with a dietitian or nutritionist before trying any nutritional plan. They can order blood tests or any other tests to check for any sensitivities and work out what will be best for you.

Chapter Thirty-Seven: Medication

Hippocrates was believed to have said: "Natural forces within us are the true healers of disease." So perhaps we do have it within us to cure our ills. This isn't to say that we couldn't use a little help from time to time, but what if the method proves to be more of a hindrance than a help?

At some time during the first few years after my diagnosis, I was prescribed medication. My memory of this isn't clear, but there are reasons for that. I may have been prescribed amitriptyline in those early years. According to Health Navigator, this is a tricyclic antidepressant, but it is also used to treat some nerve pain and prevent migraines. I've had migraines since I was eight years old, so it is very possible I was given it for this reason more than depression. Tricyclic antidepressants are prescribed for severe depression.

My anxiety attacks were more of an issue and I believe my doctor may have prescribed something to ease those symptoms.

When I was living in Whangarei, I was unemployed for a few months. Social Welfare/Income Support, which was responsible for paying the unemployment benefit, and the New Zealand Employment Service, which registered people as looking for work, were two separate entities.

At the time, the government introduced schemes very similar to one introduced in the early years of Social Security where jobseekers were sent out to work for their benefit. One such scheme was known as Taskforce Green, which had beneficiaries doing environmental-type work. The other was called Community Taskforce, which had people with administrative-type skills out doing community work in offices, and I was sent to work at a high school.

The day I was supposed to start work, I had a massive anxiety attack. While my memory of what happened is unclear, I remember going to see a doctor who gave me diazepam, otherwise known as Valium. This was supposed to calm my nerves. Enough that I did eventually get to the school.

I did not take diazepam again during my time at this job. Some years later, I was again prescribed this medication by a GP. At my lowest point, I considered taking an overdose of those pills.

I now refuse to take any kind of anti-depressant which is why I believe I have blocked out much of my experience with this type of medication. It is not so much that I don't think they will do any good, but more that I want to avoid the temptation should I get to such a low point again.

My concerns come from a few sources. Back when I was twenty-one-years-old, I began watching a soap opera set in a hospital. It was New Zealand produced and many of the actors who performed in it were those I had recognised from various local television productions or locally made films. Which was one of the reasons I began watching the show.

In one of the plots, a boy had been having problems at home and had taken an overdose of what I think was an analgesic, or painkiller. The overdose caused organ failure and he died.

My parents often took analgesics. Usually up to four times or eight tablets a day but in my father's case, more than that. Every day. My mother was not so bad, although now due to some age-related problems she experiences a lot of pain.

I can recall before my father's cancer diagnosis, when doctors were trying to figure out what was wrong, one of the questions they asked was how many of a particular painkiller he was taking per day. They seemed very concerned when told he had been taking the same dose for years.

For me, it almost felt like he had come to be dependent on this medication. Couple that with the idea that some people begin to build up a resistance to certain medications and I worried.

I do tend to be a bit of a worrywart when it comes to this type of issue. Having had suicidal ideations many times throughout the years, I try to avoid situations where it can make those feelings worse. I am also morally against narcotics (even some which can be legally prescribed), mostly out of a fear of breaking any kind of law. I am the proverbial 'goody-two-shoes'.

I have been prescribed other anti-depressants, including fluoxetine (Prozac). I did take that for a while but stopped taking it. I now refuse any anti-depressants.

Like some others I have talked to, I found that the medication had side effects that were, in essence, unwelcome. I would feel like a 'zombie' the next day. Sleepy and not 'all there'. Some medications took away my ability to think clearly, leaving me with fogginess in the brain. Others have reported the same feeling.

Do not misunderstand. I am not saying no one should take medication. This is my personal choice and what I feel comfortable with.

Some years ago, I worked for a company that had among its many clients a distributor of herbal products. I got to know the owners of this small business very well and became very interested in their products.

One of the more interesting things they told me was that many of the pharmaceutical medications today, while treating the symptoms of one problem, may also cause symptoms for another problem.

The one thing I should emphasise is that these claims were at that time were not backed up with facts and I did not follow up on these. However, this is not to say that there is no basis at all to such claims.

I have since read a lot of 'conspiracy theories' about how pharmaceutical companies are only out to make money and will tout the benefits of certain medications while playing down any problems with them. Some even suggest that these companies will only publish results of successful trials but will not publish the results of the unsuccessful trials. This may introduce some sample bias on the part of the company, or the researcher employed to undertake these trials.

In some of my research, I came across an account of a university professor who was studying the effects of anti-depressants (Hari, 2018). The professor requested data from drug companies on the results of trials of one particular medication and what he found was concerning – a large number of patients did not respond to the medication, but the company claimed the trials were successful, even though the success rate was around ten per cent.

As a trained journalist, I try to be objective and see both sides of an argument. In the United States, there are very strict regulations and studies have to be conducted to prove those claims before the Food and Drug Administration will allow such products to be released to the market.

Here in New Zealand, we have the New Zealand Medicine and Medical Devices Safety Authority (Medsafe), a Ministry of Health governed body which regulates medicines, medical devices and any foods or cosmetics developed for therapeutic use. They approve these products so they can be sold and continue to monitor for any adverse reactions in patients and handle complaints.

Many medications list certain side effects and anyone taking such a path should know what these side effects are and discuss them with their doctor.

The pharmaceutical industry, as it is today, had its beginnings in the mid to late-19th century. There are varied stories of apothecaries, dating back even further, but as an industry it began to emerge around 1870.

There are probably hundreds of stories of so-called 'snake-oil' salesmen, or as they were often called, quacks, travelling up and down the country, mostly in the United States, selling the latest 'miracle cures'. It would be natural to believe that the emerging pharmaceutical industry back then would be the equivalent of the snake-oil salesman. However, the work of the likes of biologist Alexander Fleming, who discovered penicillin in 1928, and Marie Curie, whose research in radioactivity led to the development of the x-ray, were hardly what could be termed quackery.

With the rise of huge corporate entities like Bayer, Glaxo SmithKline, Novartis, Pfizer, to name a few, there was an initial backlash against 'natural medicine'.

I once had a conversation with someone who told me that essentially the base of most pharmaceuticals is chemical and has very little difference from breaking any plant or food down to its most basic chemical composition. This is highly debatable. The opposite view of this is that anything in its more natural form is better.

Most people are aware that when a new drug is developed, it has to be put through a series of stringent trials to prove it can do what it has been developed to do. Usually this means testing on the patients who would benefit from this drug.

In these trials, the subjects are usually separated into two groups. One group is given the drug, the other a sugar pill, otherwise known as a placebo. Each member of each group is monitored carefully for any adverse reactions over the course of the trial. Neither group knows whether they have been given the drug or the placebo. This is known as the blind test. When the researcher conducting the trial also has no idea who has the drug and who has the placebo, this is called the double-blind test.

However, there is also something known as the placebo effect. There are various theories which suggest that it can be a case of 'mind over matter' in that a person undergoing the trial is convinced that the drug they have been given will do what the researcher tells them it will do. Whether they have been given the real drug or the sugar pill is irrelevant. This can skew results and may, in essence, invalidate them. It depends on how strongly they believe it.

In the field of psychology, researchers are required to follow certain guidelines. They must first have an idea for research before making a prediction, otherwise known as a hypothesis. What this means is that their theories need to be able to be tested, and either able to be proved or disproved. However, the results of their research cannot just be taken at face value. It also must be tested by their peers. The same should be true of pharmaceuticals.

Some people who have been on anti-depressants long-term have reported that their dosage has had to be increased. While this is not true for all taking medications, it does raise a few questions.

Do certain drugs lose their efficacy over time? When we look at antibiotics, it does seem possible. However, this may also be a case of viruses becoming more resistant to those antibiotics rather than the drugs losing their efficacy.

One thing that needs to be pointed out is that there is a perception about anti-depressants that those who need them are 'weak', or 'crazy'. This is another of those myths of depression that no one really wants to address. In my case, as above, it is not a matter of weakness. I just plain don't like them.

In some ways, the fact that people believe taking medication for a psychological problem is a sign of weakness is as much a fault of education as it is culture. I mentioned earlier that while more women are diagnosed with depression than men, that could be because women are more likely to seek help. Some suggest that it is because women are more emotional than men, so are more susceptible to such things. Why, then, are more men dying by suicide?

Dr Ellen McGrath suggests that depression might be seen as a 'weakness of will' instead of a medical or psychological illness. Perhaps this also comes down to the perception from some that depression is not 'real' (McGrath, 2016).

Pride is certainly a factor - the idea that we can 'handle this ourselves' without help.

Dr McGrath suggests patients look at their situation. If, for instance, they have difficulty sleeping, leading to a decreased ability to function, medication may help. If a patient is exhibiting self-destructive behaviour, this may be another reason to look at medication.

Ultimately, the decision is the patient's. Doctors may recommend certain drugs, but patients - or at least those who are reasonably self-aware - know whether medication is right for them.

However, it is also important for the doctor to check your medical history in case there are any negative interactions with anything else. For instance, one of the people I interviewed for their story was prescribed an anti-depressant that in some cases is known for increasing the risk of suicidal thoughts. As she related, she had already had two episodes prior to being given the drug and questioned why she had been prescribed it in the first place.

Medications and Side Effects

The Mayo Clinic has a list of some drugs used to treat depression. This is not meant to be a deterrent to medication, just to inform. These, along with some side effects (www.drugs.com), are:

- Selective serotonin reuptake inhibitors (SSRIs)
  - Fluoxetine
    - Hives/itching
    - Restlessness
    - Chills or fever (less common)
    - Joint or muscle pain
  - Paroxetine (Paxil, Paxeva)
    - Acid or sour stomach
    - Belching
    - Decreased appetite

- - Sleepiness
  - Stomach discomfort
- Sertraline (Zoloft)
  - Diarrhoea
  - Dizziness
  - Dyspepsia
  - Fatigue
  - Insomnia
  - Nausea
  - Headache
- Citalopram (Celexa)
  - Problems concentrating, memory problems
  - Headache
  - Drowsiness
  - Dry mouth
  - Insomnia
  - Weight changes
- Escitalopram (Lexapro)
  - Diarrhoea
  - Drowsiness
  - Headache
  - Insomnia
  - Nausea
- Serotonin and norepinephrine reuptake inhibitors (SNRIs)
  - Duloxetine (Cymbalta)
    - Constipation
    - Diarrhoea
    - Dizziness
    - Drowsiness
    - Fatigue
    - Hypersomnia
    - Insomnia
    - Nausea

- Sedated state
- Headache
- Venlafaxine (Effexor XR)
  - Asthenia (abnormal weakness or lack of energy)
  - Constipation
  - Dizziness
  - Drowsiness
  - Headache
  - Insomnia
  - Nausea
  - Nervousness
  - Anorexia
  - Decreased appetite
  - Diaphoresis (sweating)
- Desvenlafaxine (Pristiq, Khedezla)
  - Constipation
  - Dizziness
  - Drowsiness
  - Insomnia
  - Nausea
  - Decreased appetite
- Levomilnacipran (Fetzima)
  - Nausea
  - Orthostatic hypotension

- Atypical Anti-depressants
  - Trazodone
    - Blurred vision
    - Dizziness
    - Drowsiness
    - Headache
    - Nausea
    - Vomiting
  - Mirtazapine (Remeron)
    - Severe sedation

- Constipation
- Drowsiness
- Increased serum cholesterol
- Weight gain
- Fatigue
- Insomnia
- Increased appetite
- Decreased appetite
  - Vortioxetine (Trintellix)
    - Diarrhoea
    - Nausea
  - Vilazodone (Viibryd)
    - Diarrhoea
    - Nausea
  - Bupropion (Wellbutrin, Aplenzin)
    - Insomnia
    - Nausea
    - Pharyngitis (sore throat)
    - Weight loss
    - Constipation
    - Dizziness
    - Headache

- Tricyclic Anti-depressants – Common side effects are not listed
  - Imipramine (Tofranil)
  - Nortriptyline (Pamelor)
  - Amitriptyline
  - Doxepin
  - Desipramine (Norpramin)
- Monoamine Oxidase Inhibitors (MAOIs) – these may be prescribed when other medications don't work, but it sounds like a last resort as they have pretty serious interactions with some foods and other medications
  - Tranylcypromine (Parnate) – common side effects not listed

- Phenelzine (Nardil)
  - Chills
  - Cold sweats
  - Dizziness
  - Trembling
  - shakiness
- Isocarboxazid (Marplan)
  - Dizziness
  - Headache

These are by no means all the possible side effects. In all instances, there are less common side effects, and in some cases, not enough information is available on various incidences where patients have reported side effects.

Note that some of the above listed medications may not be available in New Zealand or may be given a different name. It's always best to get advice from your doctor.

Chapter Thirty-Eight: Pets

There is an advertisement that sometimes plays on New Zealand television. It's for a retirement village. In the ad, one of the staff is trying to encourage an elderly lady, Mary, to join in activities or just socialise with others in the community, but the lady is reluctant. The caregiver notices several photographs of cats as she leaves. In the next scene, Mary is being taken in a wheelchair to a common room where the viewer is shown a poster saying the retirement home is getting a cat and residents can choose it. In the next scene, Mary is once again in her room but spots a kitten chasing something in the hallway. She wants to see the kitten but realises she has to use her walking frame. She goes out to the common room to find another resident playing with the kitten. In the final scene, Mary is out in the garden, chatting to someone. She looks happy and animated.

While it is clearly a scripted scenario, it demonstrates something that mental health professionals have been advocating for years. Pets not only make great companions, but they also can provide huge benefits for those with mental health conditions.

Sigmund Freud may have realised this and there is a story, unproven, that he may have been working on such a theory around the time of his death.

An article in *Psychology Today* (Latham, 2011) mentions that Freud would have his two dogs sitting beside him during therapy sessions. He apparently also felt they had a special sense for judging character, allowing them to alert him when a patient was feeling particularly stressed.

Toward the end of his life, Freud was diagnosed with oral cancer. It probably stemmed from his habit of smoking several cigars throughout the day. He had surgery in which part of his jaw was removed. The result left him in terrible pain.

According to the story, during his last days, Freud found comfort in the company of his furry companions and began to notice how they helped relieve some of the psychological stress of his condition. So much that he supposedly began writing a paper on the topic. However, Freud died before the paper could be completed or published.

His observations and theories did not go unnoticed, and it is well-documented that pets make a significant difference in the wellbeing of someone who is struggling with mental illness. There have also been studies on how pets can sense when a person is about to have a seizure or is unwell.

A blog post on the website for The Anxiety and Depression Association of America states that some pet owners reported improvements in their mental health (Feldman).

Studies have also shown that pets and therapy animals help alleviate symptoms of stress, anxiety and depression as well as helping reduce feelings of social isolation.

It is possible that Freud knew that pets, or specifically in his case, dogs, can have a calming influence (Latham, 2011). Recent research backs this up, reporting that petting a dog helps reduce stress levels.

It is possible that animals have been used in therapeutic interventions for more than 200 years. Mention is made in an article of the York Retreat (Pereira & Fonte, 2018), an institute for the mentally disturbed in England, whereby animals were brought in to assist with therapy. This institution was established by the Society of Friends (Quakers), and opened in 1796. Inmates were treated with compassion, rather than violent beatings as other institutions were known for (History of York). The Retreat, as it is now known, is still in operation and works with the national health service in England.

Pet Partners is an organisation based in Washington State in the United States and has been in operation since 1977, although it was known as the Delta Society. It is considered a leader in demonstrating the benefits of animal-assisted therapy, activities and education in the United States (petpartners.com).

One of the organisation's founders, Dr Leo Bustad, is widely credited with introducing the term 'human-animal bond'.

Unfortunately, animal-assisted therapy is not as widely known in New Zealand but enquiries can be made through the SPCA or the Aotearoa New Zealand Association of Social Workers.

In my personal experience, I have had cats most of my life. When I was seven, my father brought home a kitten. The kitten had been part of a litter born at the warehouse where he worked. I'd begged him for it. That cat lived 14 years, and it wasn't long before I begged to be allowed another one.

In 2018, after about eight years without a pet, I was given one for my birthday. People began to notice a difference in my demeanour. I was calmer. Yes, I would talk to the cat, but doing so helped ease my loneliness and isolation.

The following are some other examples I can use to illustrate what a difference it can make:

I suffer from migraines. They can be frequent and often very painful. Twenty years ago, I was living on my own but had a cat. I was sent home from work with a bad migraine and went to bed. My cat must have sensed I was feeling unwell as she got up on the bed, curled up with my arm around her and went to sleep. This was not a cat that was known to enjoy that kind of closeness.

The cat I have now is a snuggler. As a kitten, she loved to sleep on my chest, and still likes cuddles in the mornings. There is nothing better or more calming than stroking soft fur and hearing a gentle purr.

Pets provide a sense of companionship. There are also many

other benefits, including calming anxiety and stress or encouraging people to get out, whether it's taking a dog for a walk, or meeting like-minded others.

Dr Taylor Chastain is National Director of Field Relations at Pet Partners.

Taylor has a Bachelor's degree in Psychology and a Master's degree in mental health counselling. She also obtained a Doctorate of Philosophy in research psychology where her research focused on the human-animal bond during times of human crisis and trauma recovery.

She also has eight dogs of her own - many of whom are registered or retired therapy animals.

"I'm passionate about promoting the standardisation and professionalisation of animal-assisted interventions," she says (Chastain, 2019)

Taylor states that in her own work she has anecdotal evidence that can prove these benefits.

"Pets often become a crucial part of the family system, allowing for a healthy connection that mediates many of life's challenging emotions, such as depression and anxiety."

Pet Partners doesn't just work with dogs. The organisation registers nine different species of therapy animal including cats, horses, rabbits, birds, guinea pigs, rats and even miniature pigs and llamas.

"Each of these species has different traits that position them to offer a unique benefit to a wide variety of people in the therapy animal setting."

There is a huge difference between having a service animal for anxiety, or in some cases Post Traumatic Stress Disorder, and using animal-assisted interaction for therapy.

Taylor says a therapy animal "would be trained and owned typically by its handler and the team would then go into facilities and visit for short periods with people who can benefit from the power of the human-animal bond."

In New Zealand, we often hear stories of people bringing

animals into rest homes or hospitals, as mentioned in the advertisement at the beginning of this chapter. These appear to be very effective in helping the elderly or the sick.

A study was conducted involving patients with Major Depressive Disorder who adopted a pet in an "attempt to increase response and remission rates" (Pereira & Fonte, 2018).

Of the 80 patients in the study, less than half took up the challenge. The focus was on patients who had between nine and 15 months of combined pharmacological therapy without remission.

The inclusion of pets did make a significant difference in their lives. However, the study did have its limitations in that the researchers state comparison with other studies was not possible due to its unique design and lack of other studies in that area.

The researchers note that pets can fulfil one of the basic human needs – touch, saying it releases oxytocin in the body. Oxytocin is a neuropeptide which helps in social bonding, among other things. Caring for a pet also helps reduce cortisol.

As we know from the causes chapter, stress can cause an increase in cortisol, which is known to lead to both physiological and psychological issues.

Taylor says there have been similar studies in which interactions with pets has led to a number of positive health benefits.

"In therapy animal work specifically, studies have shown that interaction with therapy animals leads to decreased stress and anxiety, increased social interaction, reduced perceptions of physical pain and even in faster healing for people who are recovering from an illness or medical procedure.

There are news stories on the work Pet Partners do via their website: **https://petpartners.org/about-us/news/.**

While not every person will be comfortable with having a pet, it is an option to consider in managing depression. Bear in mind that if you live in a rental property, some landlords may refuse to allow pets. In this instance, it is always best to talk this over with your doctor or therapist to see what avenues you can explore. You can also discuss your situation with your property manager as they may be willing to negotiate. It may even help getting your doctor to write a letter explaining your needs.

Chapter Thirty-Nine: Coping Strategies

The first thing to remember when you are not feeling your best is that you are not alone. You are not the only person in the world to feel this way or have this illness. Your experience, however, is unique to you. No one, not even another person with depression, can walk a mile in your shoes.

I have explored various things like nutrition, fitness, medication, pets. There are some other things you can do that are not necessarily to do with routines, but just some points of advice that I have found helpful.

1.   Acceptance

Accept that you have depression. Avoid denial. Accept that there will be days when you feel like you are on a high and other days where you will feel as low as you can be. Neither situation is wrong.

Do not let others tell you that you 'shouldn't feel this way'. Ask yourself if they would tell a person with a visible disability the same thing. No one has the right to tell you that you have no right to be unhappy.

2.   Understanding

Not everyone is going to be understanding of your situation. Sadly, this occurs in all things. When people try to dismiss mental illness, in a lot of cases, it is because of a lack of understanding.

While there have been some incredible breakthroughs by medical experts in this area, remember that it was not so long ago that people with all kinds of mental illness were locked up in mental institutions. Unfortunately, there are some who still feel that way, despite overwhelming medical evidence that those with some mental health problems are fully capable of leading independent lives.

I have already mentioned this, but it is worth repeating. There have been several multiple fatalities in shooting or other incidences of violence around the world. In some instances, it has been stated by media that the perpetrator has had some 'mental health issues'. That may lead people to assume that all those with these problems will become violent, when that is completely untrue.

Bear in mind, as well, that there are other health conditions that can be just as easily misunderstood. Take diabetes, for instance. There are at least two known types and most people who have never had it or have never known family with it have assumed that it is due to poor diet. That is not always the case.

There are many stories on the 'net of people who have experienced prejudice because of their illnesses. Another example is arthritis. Most people assume it is something only the elderly suffer, which is completely untrue. Others are: fibromyalgia, lupus, or multiple sclerosis. There have often been news articles of young people abused for parking in disabled spaces, when they are legally entitled to, because bystanders assume that their ability to walk means they do not have a disability.

Remember that not every illness is visible.

3.   Get Out of Your Headspace

It may sound an odd thing to say, but if you are feeling down or stressed, and if you are able to, try to do something different.

Go for a walk, read a book, watch a movie on television. Do something to take your mind off what is worrying you at that point in time. Even put some music on and dance, if that is your fancy.

Develop a hobby – writing, painting, knitting, woodwork. The possibilities are endless.

If you have an understanding boss, and I know that is not always possible, tell them what is going on and let them know that you may need to take a few minutes before settling down to work again. You can always tell them that it is better for you, and for them in the long run, to be able to walk away from a stressful situation for a few minutes rather than be unproductive.

4.   Try to avoid stimulants

Whether it is illegal drugs (or herbal alternatives), alcohol, smoking or coffee, it's best to avoid these where possible. Look into natural remedies but talk to health professionals.

5.   Alternative therapies

I have already touched on this, but Yoga and Tai Chi help with anxiety. Check your local providers for classes or search your local library for DVDs if you cannot afford to attend classes.

Hypnotherapy is always an option to explore, as is meditation. There are professionals you can talk to.

6.   Don't be afraid to be honest about your illness

The one thing I have never done is lie about my depression. I refuse to.

We have so much pressure trying to be 'good' all the time: in our work and in our personal lives. If your family or your friends cannot handle you when you are not feeling your best, or your employers place certain conditions on you not 'stressing out' at work, then find a way of getting some support system in place. An employer should not be able to discriminate against you for your illness.

7.   Never let anyone invalidate your feelings

Just because someone is going through something similar to you, it does not mean that they are worse off than you.

I have heard of others experiencing depression who have been told that a friend or relative is going through another illness and they should consider themselves lucky they don't have that illness.

8.   You do not have to take on anyone else's baggage

Sometimes others want to unload on you. That's fine, but some will do it in such a way that it feels like they expect you to either find a solution for them or take on the burden of their problem yourself.

The first step to healing depression, especially if it stems from something from your family's past, is recognising that you do not have to take on the baggage from your parents. Let them deal with their own issues. They are not yours.

9.   Some people will continue to deny that depression is real.

It is inevitable that you will meet someone who will dismiss your illness or try to tell you that it's your imagination. Sometimes the person who does that is someone you trust, like a parent, or a friend.

While you can try to educate that person on the impact of depression, it will be, sadly, like talking to a brick wall. You are not going to change their mind, even with the facts presented in front of them.

Unfortunately, if you're a minor and your parent is the one denying your depression, it may impact your ability to get the help you need. Try to adopt some of the management strategies already laid out in this book until such time as you can seek professional help without needing their approval. Or talk to your GP and explain the situation. Perhaps they can intervene on your behalf.

Section Six:
Advice For Those Who Support Someone With Depression

It is never easy living with someone who has depression or trying to be there for them. However, it's important to try to see things from their perspective.

When we are feeling down, we need support and understanding; not to be told of things we 'should' be doing.

Here is a list of things that should not be said to someone with depression.

Chapter Forty: What Not To Say

Family and friends can be very well-meaning and say things that, to someone with depression and/or anxiety can actually be harmful, not to mention, hurtful. Some of these are from anecdotes while others have come from my own experience.

Get Over It

If it were that simple, this book would not have been written. This has to be the most harmful and insensitive phrase a person can say to someone with depression. It usually comes from a place of ignorance.

Depression is not something you can just 'get over'. It is not like the common cold. It is impossible to just go to bed, sleep it off and be suddenly cured. It would be the same as saying it to someone with Multiple Sclerosis, which is one of those diseases that has its good days and bad days.

Other People Are Worse Off

As opposed to what? There are different scales of 'worse off'. Yes, people are starving in Africa, or there are wars in the Middle East, or wherever the current conflict is, but the important thing to remember is when we are in a full depressive episode, we do not really care what other people are going through.

The one thing I have always felt that depression can be a very selfish illness. It only allows us to think and feel about what we are going through at that point in time. Our perspective becomes very narrow so we can only focus on that space at that moment. We don't want to hear about our best friend's cousin's neighbour's sister who is also going through a rough time.

Calm Down

Not everyone who has depression has anxiety and not everyone who has anxiety has depression. There are times, however, when a depressive episode can bring on an attack of anxiety. When we have such an episode, the very last thing we need to hear from someone is 'calm down'.

Again, this has to do with our ability to focus. We simply cannot do that. Our worldview is completely skewed. There are various physical symptoms that accompany these episodes, from a feeling of intense pressure to vertigo. Telling someone who is experiencing these symptoms to 'calm down' is pretty much like waving a red flag at a bull.

Similarly, our moods can vary, leading sometimes to outbursts.

Grow Up

There have been times when I have been treated like a child, or spoken down to, as if my inability to handle stress in my worst moments is considered something childish. I get angry and upset but that does not mean I am acting childish.

It boils down to the fact that I am feeling very overwhelmed. I need understanding, not condescension.

Stop Crying

Believe it or not, crying is the best thing I can do to help relieve the pressure and calm myself down. It's a way to release bottled-up emotions. Some might get angry and/or violent.

This is not to say that getting angry or violent toward someone is a healthy way to release those emotions. If you feel that way, one strategy I was told was to throw something. It could be something as simple as throwing a tennis ball against the wall of the house, or whatever building you're in. Let that tension out.

Come Over Here and Get A Hug

Human touch is very important in depressive episodes, but we need to feel that someone cares enough to make the effort. At times, we may be in such a state that we can't physically move. It has been said that it takes strength just to even get out of bed during these episodes. So, when someone tells us to come to them to get a hug, although they are well-meaning, it's like asking us to climb Mt Everest.

Sometimes all we really need is for someone to hold our hand.

You're Too Uptight

We know there are times when we are too tightly wound. We don't need to be told that.

When someone has a mental illness, there are certain times when routine is very important. Change can be a little overwhelming. That sometimes means that we are a little too rigid, a little too set in our ways. That does not mean it is wrong or that we cannot cope with change. We can, but it just takes us a little longer than everyone else to find our feet.

You're Making A Mountain Out of a Molehill/Overreacting

In moments of anxiety, what looks like an overreaction to someone else is actually quite normal to us. The point is, just because someone else can handle stress better than we can, does not mean that our reaction is over the top or that we are creating a mountain out of a molehill.

Try Prayer

I have been preached at and told to pray to God, Jesus or whomever to fix my problems. Religion is not for everyone and at times it can make a person feel extremely uncomfortable. Talking, however, is good for the spirit. Even if it means raging at the sky or whatever.

Everybody Gets Stressed

So what? Maybe everyone does get stressed at certain points in their life, but we are not talking about everyone else. This is worth repeating. Depression is a selfish illness. When I am depressed it is all: 'me, me, me'. I don't care about anyone else.

Again?

There are times when we get tired of going through depressive episodes ourselves. The last thing we need from our families and friends is to see them roll their eyes, sigh and act as if our illness is a major inconvenience to them. Or that they are tired and annoyed at going through this 'again'.

Stop Being So Negative/Change Your Mindset

For some of us, we are our own worst critics and it is extremely difficult to change a mindset when the negative voice is at times the loudest voice we hear. It really is not that easy to change a way of thinking that has dominated your thoughts for a very long time. Telling a person with depression they are too negative is very unhelpful, and in many ways, just as damaging. It is very similar to the 'get over it'. Even if that change of mind is achieved, it does not cure the depression.

You Don't Know What Stress Is

We define stress as something such as, trying to pay a mortgage, raising a family. Some people tend to forget that there are different types of stress. As in an earlier chapter, stress can occur from tragic situations, but we can also experience stress from events such as a wedding, or a family reunion.

There is positive and negative stress. There is the kind of stress that can get the blood or the adrenaline pumping and there is the kind of stress that can make us feel like we have an elephant on our chest, making it very difficult for us to breathe.

Telling someone they have no idea what stress is just makes them feel like their problems are unimportant.

Get Help

Not everyone has this available. Getting help would be wonderful, but there are some places where the health system just cannot cope with mental health issues. When money is a factor, it can be a huge barrier to getting that help.

There have been times when I have considered support groups, but transport was an issue. When I lived in Auckland, I contacted one such support group, only to be told it met in an area that I could only get to by bus. It would finish late at night, leaving me to catch a late bus back home, in an area where I did not feel safe, which caused anxiety. Auckland is not a safe place for a woman travelling on her own on public transport.

Smile

I have seen this in forums on customer service, where a cashier is told to smile. I realise that in this field of work, the customer is everything, and management often has a policy that the customer service person must appear to be at their best at all times, but this is not always possible.

Again, this is something we don't want to hear. To add to that, the 'Smile, it's not that bad'. To that I say, 'how would you know?' Sometimes it is that bad and we can barely muster up a grimace.

Please remember that you do not always know what someone else is going through, so try not to be judgemental.

You're successful/rich. You have no reason to be unhappy

There are dozens of stories of successful people who have battled depression.

Firstly, the idea that because someone is successful and/or a celebrity, they have no reason to be unhappy is complete ignorance. Being a celebrity is hugely stressful. They have no privacy.

A few years ago a woman named Charlotte Dawson, a former model and television presenter, was found dead in her apartment in Australia. Her death was ruled suicide. There had been reports of trolls on Twitter leaving offensive messages for Charlotte. She had had some troubles in the years leading up to her death.

You're able to get out and about, you're not lying in bed unable to move – you don't have depression

This is actually related to another chronic illness I have. Let me make something very clear. There are varying degrees of depression, just like there are varying degrees of other illnesses. Just because someone is out of bed and able to do things, go to work, etc., does not mean they don't have depression. Before someone says something so judgemental, perhaps they need to go and do some research.

Also, do not assume that because you suffer from something similar, you know everything and can say such things to another person with the same illness.

Stop Living in the Past

I have explored where my depression comes from and yet people believe that I am living in the past because of it. If someone has an illness or disability caused by something that happened to them long ago, they at least know the source of that illness.

Studies show that certain events through our lives can have lasting physical or emotional effects. Letting go of past hurts is not as easy as some people make it out to be, and sometimes the only way to do that is to understand where it comes from. To put it simply, if you do not explore where or how the depression began, you would not be able to move on. Also, by not dealing with what caused it, if something happens later on, the depression could return (Harvard, 2009).

Why Don't You ...?

While this is well-meaning, we do not need advice on how to deal with our depression from someone who has not been there. Sometimes we also don't want to hear it from someone who <u>has</u> been there.

I have had people advise me on what jobs I should be going for, when they think that I should be going for jobs that are lower than my qualifications. I know what I can handle. They don't.

Similarly, I have had well-meaning advice from others on what I eat, whether I should be getting therapy and so on.

Last Word

The final thing I would say to anyone is try to remember that the more we are told the word 'should', the more likely we are to dig our heels in and refuse. Sometimes we need to be left alone to deal with it in our own time. That may mean we don't want to spend time with others and just need to be alone. That is not always a bad thing.

Just because we choose to be alone at certain times, does not mean we are planning on drastic action. Don't demand that we open up and talk to you either. Let us come to you.

Above all, listen.

Websites

- Articles on mental health – Psychology Today - **https://www.psychologytoday.com/nz**
- Beyond Blue support group - **https://www.facebook.com/groups/groupbeyondblue/**
- Depression.org.nz – **http://depression.org.nz**
- Mental Health Foundation - **https://www.mentalhealth.org.nz/**
- Ministry of Health - **https://www.health.govt.nz/**
- National Institute of Mental Health - **https://www.nimh.nih.gov/index.shtml**
- New Zealand Association of Counsellors - **http://www.nzac.org.nz/code_of_ethics.cfm**.
- Pet Partners - **https://petpartners.org/**
- World Health Organisation - **https://www.who.int/**

BIBLIOGRAPHY

Ability Magazine. *Abraham Lincoln*. Retrieved from:
  https://www.abilitymagazine.com/abe_story.html

Abrams, Allison. 5 Depression Myths We Need to Stop
  Believing Today. *Psychology Today*. Posted February 1,
  2018. Retrieved from:
  https://www.psychologytoday.com/us/blog/nurturi
  ng-self-compassion201802/5-depression-myths-we-
  need-stop-believing-today, January 2019.

American Psychiatric Association. *Diagnostic and Statistical
  Manual of Mental Disorders* (DSM5), 2013.

Diagnostic and Statistical Manual of Mental Disorders
  (DSM5), 2013.

Australian Bureau of Statistics. *Mental and Behavioural
  Conditions. National Health Survey: First Results 2017-18.*
  Released December 2018, retrieved from:
  http://www.abs.gov.au/ausstats/abs@.nsf/Lookup/b
  y%20Subject/4364.0.55.001~2017-
  18~Main%20Features~Mental%20and%20behavioural
  %20conditions~70, April 2019.

Beatty, Jack. President Coolidge's Burden. *The Atlantic*.
  December 2003. Retrieved from:
  https://www.theatlantic.com/magazine/archive/2003
  /12/president-coolidges-burden/303175/

Beyond Blue Support Service. Statistics. Retrieved from:
  https://www.beyondblue.org.au/media/statistics,
  April 2019.

Black Dog Institute. *What is Depression*. Retrieved from:
https://www.blackdoginstitute.org.au/clinical-
resources/depression/what-is-depression

Bloodworth-Thomason, Linda, Place, Mary Kay. Mad Dogs
and Servicemen. *M*A*S*H*. 3:13, 1974. 20th Century
Fox.

Borchard. Therese. 9 Steps to Treat Depression Naturally.
Everyday Health. October 2015. Retrieved from:
https://www.everydayhealth.com/columns/therese-
borchard-sanity-break/steps-treat-depression-
naturally/, October 2018.

Bowler, Peter J. *Darwin: Off the Record*. Duncan Baird
Publishers, London. 2010.

Boyle, Chelsea. New Zealand suicides highest since records
began. *NZ Herald*. January 22, 2019. retrieved from:
https://www.nzherald.co.nz/nz/news/article.cfm?c_i
d=1&objectid=12112773, January 2019.

Breckenridge, Carol. Leading Churchill Myths - The Myth of
the 'Black Dog'. *International Churchill Society*. Summer
2012. Retrieved from: https://winstonchurchill.org
/publications/finest-hour/finest-hour-155/the-myth-
of-the-black-dog/

Brown, Gregory K.; Karlin, Bradley E.; Trockel, Mickey;
Gordienko, Maria; Yesavage, Jerry; and Barr Taylor, C.
Effectiveness of Cognitive Behavioral Therapy for
Veterans with Depression and Suicidal Ideation.
Archives of Suicide Research. 20:677-682, 2016. Retrieved
from:
https://www.tandfonline.com/doi/full/10.1080/1381
1118.2016.1162238 June 2019.

Burton, Robert. *The Anatomy of Melancholy*. First edition 1621.

Campbell AK, Matthews SB. Darwin Diagnosed. *Biological
Journal of the Linnean Society*. 2015.

Campbell, Archie. *Hee Haw*. (CBS 1969-71).

Careers. *Psychiatrist*. Retrieved from: https://www.careers.
govt.nz/jobs-database/health-and-community/health

/psychiatrist/how-to-enter-the-job, July 2019.

Carlson, Neil R., Buskist, William. The Treatment of Mental Disorders. *Psychology: The Science of Behaviours.* Allyn and Bacon. 1997.

Chastain, Dr Taylor. *Pet Partners.* Email interview July 2019

Christianson, Gale E. *Isaac Newton.* Oxford University Press. 2005.

Christ's College Cambridge. *History.* Retrieved from: https://www.christs.cam.ac.uk/history-christs-college

Dewey, Catilin. A stunning map of depression rates around the world. *Washington Post.* November 7, 2013. Retrieved from: https://www.washingtonpost.com/news/worldviews/wp/2013/11/07/a-stunning-map-of-depression-rates-around-the-world/?noredirect=on&utm_ter&utm_term=.48740aba3987. April, 2018.

Diamond, Stephen A (Ph.D). Is Depression A Disease? in Evil Deeds. *Psychology Today.* September 01, 2008. https://www.psychologytoday.com/us/blog/evil-deeds. Retrieved August 2018. Used with permission.

Dictionary.com. *Definition of Sadness.* Retrieved from: https://www.dictionary.com/browse/sadness, January 2019

Dresden, Danielle. What is the hippocampus? *Medical News Today.* Retrieved from: https://www.medicalnewstoday.com/articles/313295.php, April 2019

Drugs.com. *Drug Side Effects.* Retrieved from: https://www.drugs.com/sfx/ July 2019.

Dunn, Andrea, L.; Trivedi, Madhukar, H.; Kampert, James B.; Clark, Camillia G.; and Chambliss, Heather O. Exercise Treatment for Depression: Efficacy and Dose Response. *American Journal of Preventive Medicine.* 28. 1-8. 10.1016/j.amepre.2004.09.003.

Farber, Neil. The Truth About the Law of Attraction: It Doesn't Exist. *Psychology Today.* September 2016.

Retrieved from: https://www.psychologytoday.com/ blog/the-blame-game/201609/the-truth-about-the-law -attraction. June 2019.

Fallis, Jordan. Studies Reveal Taking Probiotics Reduces Risk of Anxiety and Depression. *Healthy Holistic Living.* November 10, 2017. Retrieved from: https://www.healthy-holistic-living.com/studies-reveal-taking-probiotics-reduces-risk-anxiety-depression/. April 2019.

Feldman, Steven. Alleviating anxiety, stress and depression with the pet effect. *Adaa.org.* https://adaa.org/learn-from-us/from-the-experts/blog-posts/consumer/alleviating-anxiety-stress-and-depression-pet. Retrieved April 2019.

Firth, Joseph; Marx, Wolfgang; Dash, Sarah; Carney, Rebekah, Teasdale, Scott B.; Solmi, Marco, Stubbs, Brendon; Schuch, Felipe B. Carvalho, Andre F; Jacka, Felice and Sarris, Jerome. The Effects of Dietary Improvement on Symptoms of Depression and Anxiety: A Meta-Analysis of Randomized Controlled Trials. *Psychosomatic Medicine.* 81(3):265–280, APR 2019, retrieved from: https://insights.ovid.com/crossref?an=00006842-201904000-00007, linked from NICM at Western Sydney University, July 2019.

Firth, Joseph. Eating a healthy diet can ease symptoms of depression. *News and Events. NICM.* 6 February 2019. Retrieved from: https://westernsydney.edu.au/nicm/ news/eating_a_healthy_diet_can_ease_symptoms_of_ depression, July 2019.

Freedland, Michael. *Judy Garland: The Other Side of the Rainbow.* JR Books. London. 2010.

Freud, S. (1917). Mourning and Melancholia. *The Standard Edition of the Complete Psychological Works of Sigmund Freud, Volume XIV (1914-1916): On the History of the Psycho-Analytic Movement, Papers on Metapsychology and*

Other Works.

Frost, Bob. Mark Twain: Highwater and Hell. *Biography Magazine.* 2002. Retrieved from: http://www.historyaccess.com/marktwain-histor.html.

Fulford, Robert. *An Unmoveable Beast.* National Post. August 2, 2016. Retrieved from: https://nationalpost.com/entertainment/books/ernest-hemingway-depression-anger-plagued-him-until-it-was-time-for-him-to-die. August 2019.

Ghaemi, Nassir. A Great Businessman – A Failed Leader. *Psychology Today.* September, 2012. Retrieved from: https://www.psychologytoday.com/us/blog/mood-swings/201209/great-businessman-failed-political-leader

Gilbert, Martin. *Churchill: A Life.* Pimlico. 2000. First published: William Heinemann Ltd. 1991.

Gingell, Sarah. How Your Mental Health Reaps the Benefits of Exercise. *Psychology Today.* March 22, 2018. Retrieved from: https://www.psychologytoday.com/us/blog/what-works-and-why/201803/how-your-mental-health-reaps-the-benefits-exercise. May 2018.

Glenza, Jessica. Ketamine-related drug could be 'watershed' in treating depression. *The Guardian.* March 8, 2019. Retrieved from: https://www.theguardian.com/society/2019/mar/08/new-ketamine-drug-could-be-watershed-in-treating-depression, March 2019.

Gorman, Herbert, S. Bizarre Career of a Mad French Painter; Vincent Van Gogh. A Biographical Study by Julius Meter-Graefe, Translated by John Hoiroyd Reece. Review. *New York Times.* 22 April 1923.

Grohol, John M. 7 Myths of Depression. *Psych Central.* July 2018. Retrieved from: https://psychcentral.com/blog/7-myths-of-depression/, January 2019.

Gussow, Mel. Tennessee Williams Is Dead Here At 71. *New York Times*. 26 February 1983.

Gussow, Mel. Williams Is Mourned By Friends And Others. *New York Times*. 28 February 1983.

Hari, Johann. *Lost Connections : Uncovering the Real Causes of Depression - and the Unexpected Solutions*. Bloomsbury Publishing Plc, 2018. ProQuest Ebook Central, http://ebookcentral.proquest.com/lib/massey/detail.action?docID=5242424, April 2019.

Harvard Medical School. *What Causes Depression*. Harvard Health Publishing. Published June 2009, updated April 2017. Retrieved from: https://www.health.harvard.edu/mind-and-mood/what-causes-depression 1/17, March 2019.

Hay, Louise L. *About Louise Hay*. Retrieved from: http://louisehay.com April 2019.

Hill, David. *Health Hub Project*. Palmerston North. Interview. May 2018.

Hippocrates. *Aphorisms*, vol 4, Section 6.23, p 185, Loeb Classical Library, 1923, Heraclitus, of Ephesus; Jones, W.H.S; Potter, Paul; Smith, Wesley D; Withington, E.T.

History of York.org. The Retreat. *History of York*. Retrieved from: http://www.historyofyork.org.uk/themes/georgian/the-retreat, July 2019.

Humphries, Mark. University of Nottingham. Email communication. April 2019.

Humphries, Mark. A New Prime Suspect for Depression: And the hunt for its neural causes. *The Spike*. Medium.com, May 2018. Retrieved from: https://medium.com/the-spike/a-new-prime-suspect-for-depression-4a4607a870b0, April 2019.

Kakutani, Michiko. The Legacy of Tennessee Williams. *New York Times*. 6 March 1983.

Kandola, Aaron. What are the consequences of a sedentary Lifestyle. Medical News Today. August 2018. Retrieved from: https://www.medicalnewstoday.com/articles/

3229010.php. August 2019.

King's School. History. Retrieved from:
https://www.kings.lincs.sch.uk/page/?title=The+Sch
ool+History&pid=37

Latham, Tyger. Dogs, Man's Best Therapist. *Psychology Today*.
April 8, 2011 Retrieved from:
https://www.psychologytoday.com/us/blog/therapy
-matters/201104/dogs-man-s-best-therapist, April
2019.

Liddell, Henry and Robert Scott (1980). *A Greek-English Lexicon
(Abridged Edition)*. United Kingdom: Oxford University
Press.

Longfellow, Henry Wadsworth. *The Rainy Day*. 1842. retrieved
from https://www.thoughtco.com/the-rainy-day-
quotes-2831517, January 2019.

Marano, Hara Estroff. Depression Doing the Thinking.
Psychology Today. July 1, 2001 (reviewed June 9, 2016).
Retrieved from:
https://www.psychologytoday.com/us/articles/2001
07/depression-doing-the-thinking, January 2019.

Mayo Clinic Staff. Mediterranean Diet: A heart healthy eating
plan. *Nutrition and Healthy Eating*. Mayo Clinic. June 21,
2019. Retrieved from:
https://www.mayoclinic.org/healthy-lifestyle
/nutrition-and-healthy-eating/in-
depth/mediterranean-diet/art-20047801. August 2019.

McGrath, Ellen. How to Think About Medication. *Psychology
Today*. April 1, 2002, reviewed June 9, 2016, retrieved
from: https://www.psychologytoday.com/us/
articles/200204/how-think-about-medication, April
2019.

McManus, Katherine D. What is a plant-based diet and why
should you try it? *Harvard Health Blog*. Harvard Health
Publishing. Harvard Medical School. Updated: 27
September, 2048. Retrieved from: https://www.
health.harvard.edu./blog/what-is-a-plant-based-diet

-and-why-should-you-tri-it-2018092614760.

McPherson, James, M. *Abraham Lincoln*. Oxford 2009.

Medical News. *22 Surprising Habits of People Hiding Depression*. Retrieved from: https://medical-news.org/22-surprising-habits-of-people-hiding-depression/13880/5/. August 2019.

Mental Health Foundation. UK. *Fundamental Facts about Mental Health*. Retrieved from: https://www.mentalhealth.org.uk/publications/fundamental-facts-about-mental-health-2016, March 2019.

Mental Health Foundation UK. *Suicide*. Retrieved from https://www.mentalhealth.org.uk/a-to-z/s/suicide, April 2019.

Ministry of Business and Innovation. *Counsellors and Psychologists*. Retrieved from: https://occupationoutlook.mbie.govt.nz/social-and-community/counsellors-and-psychologists/ July 2019.

Ministry of Health NZ. *Health Survey*. https://minhealthnz.shinyapps.io/nz-health-survey-2016-17-annual-data-explorer/_w_37f19f89/#!/download-data-sets retrieved March 2018

National Institute of Mental Health. *Major Depression*. Retrieved from https://www.nimh.nih.gov/health/statistics/major-depression.shtml, May 2018.

National Institute of Mental Health. *Mental Health Information Statistics on Suicide*. Retrieved from https://www.nimh.nih.gov/health/statistics/suicide.shtml, April 2019.

National Institute of Mental Health. *Prevalence of Major Depressive Episode Among Adults*. Retrieved from https://www.nimh.nih.gov/health/statistics/major-depression.shtml, April 2019.

Newton, Phil. From Mouse to Man. *Psychology Today*. Retrieved from: https://www.psychologytoday.com/intl/blog/mouse-man, March 2019.

New York Times. Special. Judy Garland, 47, Found Dead. *New York Times*. 23 June, 1969.

New York Times. Brilliant Stardom and Personal Tragedy Punctuated the Life of Marilyn Monroe. *New York Times*. 6 August 1962.

New Zealand Association of Counsellors. *Are You Thinking of Becoming A Counsellor?* Retrieved from: http://www.nzac.org.nz/want_to_be_a_counsellor.cfm July 2019.

NZ Government. *He Ara Oranga Report of the Government Inquiry into Mental Health and Addiction*. Executive Summary and Recommendations 2018. Retrieved from https://www.mentalhealth.inquiry.govt.nz, January 2019.

NZQA. *Bachelor's Degree*. Retrieved from: https://www.nzqa.govt.nz/studying-in-new-zealand/understand-nz-quals/bachelors-degree/, July 2019.

Nuno-Perez, Alvaro; Tchenio, Anna; Mameli, Manuel; Lecca, Salvatore. Lateral Habenula Gone Awry in Depression. *Frontiers in Neuroscience*. July 2018, retrieved from: https://www.frontiersin.org/articles/10.3389/fnins.2018.00485/full, April 2019.

Owlcation.com. *A Biographical Analysis of Virginia Woolf: The Impact of Mental Illness in Woolf's Life, Marriage, and Literature*. January 22, 2018. Retrieved from: https://owlcation.com/humanities/A-Biographical-Analysis-of-Virginia-Woolf-The-Influence-of-Mental-Illness-on-a-Stable-Marriage. August 2019.

Pereira, Jorge Mota and Fonte, Daniela. Pets Enhance Antidepressant Pharmacopatherapy Effects in Patients with Treatment Resistant Major Depressive Disorder. *Journal of Psychiatric Research* 104 (2018) 108–113 Retrieved from: https://www.sciencedirect.com/science/article/abs/pii/S002239561830164X?via%3Dihub July 2019.

Pet Partners. *About Us*. Retrieved from:
    https://petpartners.org/about-us/, July 2019.
Psychology Today Staff. Celebrity Meltdown. Nov 1, 1999.
    Retrieved from: https://www.psychologytoday.com
    /nz/articles/199911/celebrity-meltdown
Queensland Brain Institute. *What Are Neurotransmitters*.
    Retrieved from: https://qbi.uq.edu.au/brain/brain-
    physiology/what-are-neurotransmitters, March 2019.
Robinson, Andrew. Does Madness Enhance or Diminish
    Genius? *Psychology Today*. March, 2011.
    https://www.psychologytoday.com/us/blog/sudden-
    genius/201103/does-madness-enhance-or-diminish-
    genius
Rowling, J.K. *Harry Potter and the Prisoner of Azkaban*.
    Bloomsbury Publishing. Great Britain, 1999. paperback
    edition 2004.
Sathyanarayana Rao, M. R. Asha, B. N. Ramesh, and K. S.
    Jagannatha Rao. Understanding nutrition, depression
    and mental illnesses. *Indian Journal of Psychiatry*. Apr-
    Jun 2008, 50(2). Retrieved from US National Library of
    Medicine. https://www.ncbi.nlm.nih.gov/pmc
    /articles/PMC2738337/. May 2018.
Scaccia, Annamarya. Serotonin: What You Need to Know.
    Healthline, 2017. Retrieved from:
    https://www.healthline.com/health/mental-
    health/serotonin, March 2019.
Seladi-Schulman, Jill. Hypothalamus Overview. *Healthline*.
    March 1, 2018. Retrieved from:
    https://www.healthline.com/human-body-
    maps/hypothalamus, April 2019
Shenk, Joshua Wolf. Lincoln's Great Depression. *The Atlantic*.
    October 2005. Retrieved from:
    https://www.theatlantic.com/magazine/archive/2005
    /10/lincolns-great-depression/304247/
Singh, Anita. Churchill's black dog is a myth and he never
    suffered depression, says leading historian. *The*

Telegraph. 6 October 2018. Retrieved from
https://www.telegraph.co.uk/news/2018/10/06/
churchills-black-dog-myth-never-suffered-depression-
says-leading/. February 2019.

Society for Endocrinology. *Cortisol. You and Your Hormones.*
Retrieved from: http://www.yourhormones.info
/hormones/cortisol/ April 2019.

Sophocles. *Ajax.* Translated by Ian Johnston. Richer Resources
Publications (April 18, 2010).

Spoto, Donald. *The Kindness of Strangers: The Life of Tennessee
Williams.* The Bodley Head. London. 1985.

Stats NZ. *Census Data* Retrieved from:
http://nzdotstat.stats.govt.nz/wbos/Index.aspx?DataS
etCode=TABLECODE8021&_ga=2.33879076.44378185.1
551121266-371828101.1551121266#, February 2019, used
with permission.

Turner, Camilla. Mystery of Agatha Christie's disappearance
is solved. *The Telegraph.* 8 May 2017. Retrieved from:
https://www.telegraph.co.uk/news/2017/05/08/mys
tery-agatha-christies-disappearance-solved-author-
suggests/, January 2019.

Twain, Mark. *Autobiography of Mark Twain.* Edited by Harriet
Elinor Smith and other editors of the Mark Twain
Project. Volume 1. University of California Press. 2010.

Udobang, Wana. In Nigeria, where mental health is often
considered a 'Western' issue, people are turning to one
another for help. *Yahoo! Lifestyle.* Retrieved from:
https://www.yahoo.com/lifestyle/nigeria-mental-
health-often-considered-western-issue-people-turning-
one-another-help-202140970.html, April 2018.

Whedon, Joss. Welcome to the Hellmouth. *Buffy the Vampire
Slayer.* Episode 1. 1997. Written by Joss Whedon.
Mutant Enemy.

Wikipedia. *Abraham Lincoln.* Retrieved from:
https://en.wikipedia.org/wiki/Abraham_Lincoln

Wikipedia. *Agatha Christie*. Retrieved from:
    https://en.wikipedia.org/wiki/Agatha_Christie,
    August 2019.
Wikipedia. *Calvin Coolidge*. Retrieved from:
    https://en.wikipedia.org/wiki/Calvin_Coolidge.
Wikipedia. *Great Plague of London*. Retrieved from:
    https://en.wikipedia.org/wiki/Great_Plague_of_Lond
    on
Wikipedia. *History of Depression*. Retrieved from:
    https://en.wikipedia.org/w/index.php?title=History_
    of_depression&oldid=831971022. Last edited 23 March
    2018.
Wikipedia. *Hypochondriasis*. Retrieved from:
    https://en.wikipedia.org/wiki/Hypochondriasis,
    March 2019.
Wikipedia. Isaac Newton. Retrieved from:
    https://en.wikipedia.org/wiki/Isaac_Newton.
Wikipedia. *Judy Garland*. Retrieved from:
https://en.wikipedia.org/wiki/Judy_Garland
Wikipedia. *Mark Twain*. Retrieved from:
    https://en.wikipedia.org/wiki/Mark_Twain.
Wikipedia.org. *Tennessee Williams*. Retrieved from:
    https://en.wikipedia.org/wiki/Tennessee_Williams
Wikipedia. *Vincent van Gogh*. Retrieved from:
    https://en.wikipedia.org/wiki/Vincent_van_Gogh
Wikipedia. *Walter Bradford Cannon*. Retrieved from:
    https://en.wikipedia.org/wiki/Walter_Bradford_Can
    non, April 2019.
Wikipedia. *Winston Churchill*. Retrieved from:
    https://en.wikipedia.org/wiki/Winston_Churchill
World Health Organisation. *Depression and Other Common
    Mental Disorders*. Retrieved from:
    https://www.who.int/mental_health/management/d
    epression/prevalence_global_health_estimates/en/,
    January 2020

World Health Organisation. *Overview of Depression*. Retrieved
   from: https://www.who.int/news-room/fact-
   sheets/detail/depression, March 2019.
Yan Yang; Hao Wang; Ji Hu; Hailan Hu. Lateral habenula in
   the pathophysiology of depression. *ScienceDirect*.
   Retrieved from: https://www.sciencedirect.com
   /science/article/pii/S0959438817302908, March 2019.
Young, Philip. *Ernest Hemingway*. Encyclopaedia Britannica.
   July 2019. Retrieved from:
   https://www.britannica.com/biography/Ernest-
   Hemingway, August 2019.

www.ingramcontent.com/pod-product-compliance
Lightning Source LLC
Chambersburg PA
CBHW032103280326

41933CB00009B/739